The effects of environment on cells and tissues

The effects of environment
on cells and tissues

*Proceedings of the IX World Congress of Anatomic
and Clinical Pathology, Sydney, 13-17 October, 1975*

Editor
E. S. FINCKH

*Institute of Clinical Pathology and Medical Research,
Lidcombe, N.S.W., Australia*

Co-editor
E. CLAYTON-JONES

1976
Excerpta Medica, Amsterdam – Oxford

International Congress Series No. 384.

ISBN Excerpta Medica 90 219 0316 4
ISBN American Elsevier 0 444 15218 0

Library of Congress Cataloging in Publication Data

World Congress of Anatomic and Clinical Pathology, 9th, Sydney, 1975.
The effects of environment on cells and tissues.

(International Congress series; no. 384)
Includes index.
1. Pathology–Congresses. 2. Anatomy, Pathological–Congresses. 3. Environmentally induced diseases–Congresses. I. Finckh. E. S. II. Clayton-Jones, E. III. Title. IV. Series. [DNLM: 1. Histology–Congresses. 2. Pathology–Congresses. W3 EX89 no. 384 1975 / QZ140 W929 1975e]
RB3.W67 1975 616.07 76-3570 ISBN 0-444-15218-0 (American Elsevier)

Publisher:
Excerpta Medica
305 Keizersgracht
Amsterdam
P.O. Box 1126

Sole Distributors for the USA and Canada:
Elsevier North-Holland Inc.
52 Vanderbilt Avenue
New York, N.Y. 10017

Typeset and printed in The Netherlands by Drukkerij Hooiberg B.V., Epe

WORLD ASSOCIATION OF SOCIETIES OF PATHOLOGY
(ANATOMIC AND CLINICAL)

IX WORLD CONGRESS OF ANATOMIC AND CLINICAL PATHOLOGY

Sydney, 13—17 October, 1975

President of Honour

EDGAR F. THOMSON

Foundation President and Advisor to the Executive,
The Royal College of Pathologists of Australia

Sponsor

World Association of Societies of Pathology

Host Society

The Royal College of Pathologists of Australia

President

Peter I. A. HENDRY

Honorary Vice-Presidents
(nominated by the Congress)

J. J. ANDUJAR, D. J. JAUMAIN, R. KOURILSKY,
Wm H. McMENEMEY, T. De SANCTIS MONALDI, M. WELSCH

Honorary Vice-Presidents
(nominated by the member societies)

W. BOSTICK (U.S.A.), D. B. DORSEY (U.S.A.), O. FENNER (Federal
Republic of Germany), F. HAMPSON (United Kingdom),
G. F. KIPKIE (Canada), N. KOSAKAI (Japan), E. LEVY (Israel),
E. MURPHY STACK (Mexico), J. PINHEIRO (Brazil),
M. RAPAPORT (Argentina)

Organizing Committee

Chairman:	Peter I. A. HENDRY
Vice-Chairmen:	T. J. CONSTANCE, E. S. FINCKH
Members:	R. A. OSBORN (Secretary), E. F. THOMSON,
	F. D. WHITE, R. A. HAYES, A. E. GATENBY,
	A. J. CLARKE, W. E. L. DAVIES (Treasurer)

Scientific Programme Committee

Chairman:	Ernest S. FINCKH
Members:	S. M. BELL (Microbiology), B. H. COOMBES
	(Anatomical Pathology), K. M. MATTOCKS
	(Chemical Pathology), F. D. WHITE (Laboratory
	Organization)

Foreword

In recent years the two main aspects of pathology – the attempt to understand the nature of disease and the laboratory assessment of disease in individuals – have unfortunately tended to separate. So as to oppose this trend the Scientific Programme Committee of the IX Triennial World Congress of the World Association of Societies of Pathology decided to devise a programme which would include and mingle both aspects, in the hope that those whose everyday activities dealt mainly with the one would become better acquainted with the other.

The great current interest in the utilisation of the clinical pathology laboratory and the evaluation of its results made it easy to include in the programme material relating to testing for disease. However, because of its wide scope, it was harder to select material concerned with the basic understanding of disease. Eventually it was decided to concentrate upon a general theme, 'The Effects of Environment on Cells and Tissues', so as to emphasize the dynamic interactions that are now understood to underlie the attainment and maintenance of normality in tissues and that, when disordered, often lead to disease. This theme owes a great deal to concepts proposed by Paul Weiss, who, as biologist not pathologist, has greatly helped in understanding the complex yet comprehensible interrelationships between the various levels of organisation in bodily tissues. As his well-known diagram on the cover of this book clearly shows, nuclear components interact dynamically with components in the cell cytoplasm; cytoplasmic components react with factors outside the cell; cells grouped together as tissues react with circulating agents of both endogenous and exogenous origin and the whole body interacts with favourable and unfavourable factors in its environment.

It was felt that such a theme was particularly appropriate for the present time, having in mind current general interest in environmental conservation and the way man interacts with his environment. It would accord with present moves for environmental improvement by indicating how external factors, chemical, physical, microbiological, or even social, might adversely affect susceptible individuals. The Organising Committee of Congress considers it fortunate that such eminent speakers, many from disciplines hitherto only too rarely linked to pathology, agreed to present addresses of such wide-ranging interest and stimulating nature at the Plenary Sessions of Congress both in relation to the above theme and to 'The Clinical Laboratory'. These addresses are now presented in slightly expanded form in this volume so as to be accessible to a wider audience. It is unfortunate that limitations of space have prevented the inclusion of the many interesting and informative proffered papers on similar or unrelated topics that were also presented to Congress. However, these have already been published in abstract form (Excerpta Medica, International Congress Series No. 369) and many will no doubt be published in full elsewhere. It is greatly to be hoped that any added momentum which may have been attained at this Congress towards the integration of basic biological concepts with the everyday practice of pathology will continue, thus securing the place of pathology as the keystone in the bridge between basic biology and the understanding and control of human disease.

E. S. Finckh
Chairman, Scientific Programme Committee

Contents

4: The external environment of the body

5: The nature of tumours

6: The behaviour of tumours

7: The clinical laboratory 1975-1984

8: Accuracy assessment and target values

9: Standards in anatomic pathology

Opening address by
H.E. the Hon. Sir John Kerr

A.C., K.C.M.G., K. St.J., Q.C., Governor-General of Australia

It is a very great honour to have the opportunity, at your invitation, to open this IX World Congress of the World Association of Societies of Pathology and to address this gathering.

You are to discuss a number of highly technical matters within the field of pathology and, of course, there is nothing that I can say about such matters. The exciting thing from my point of view is the general theme which you have adopted for your Congress – 'The effect of environment on cells and tissues'.

It is a great honour for Australia and the city of Sydney to have been selected as the venue for this important congress and for the discussion of such a theme.

The Royal College of Pathologists of Australia is also greatly honoured in being the host for this truly international and highly distinguished Congress. The College has, I know, worked very hard to make the Congress a success.

As I have said, it is of great interest to me that the principal theme of this IX Triennial Congress relates to the effects of the environment on cells and tissues. Both the science of pathology and the study of the environment represent separate areas of knowledge, each of great complexity and of vast scientific and social importance. Consideration of the interaction of the two is clearly relevant to a period when communities are re-thinking their attitude to the external environment and the complexities of its effect on human beings.

Whilst considering the effects of the external environment on man and the many ways in which various external influences exert an effect on the health and development of man, it is necessary to consider also the internal environment of the human body itself. For example, one may very well need to bring one's attention to the microscopic level of the community of cells, tissues and organs which together make up the living organism. What are the environmental relationships between these cells and tissues; how do they interreact; what are the effects of one upon the other; how is equilibrium maintained or lost?

These are the searching and important questions which pathologists are able to consider, and to which they will be giving attention throughout this Congress.

As to the internal environment of the human body itself, I must leave all the technical questions to you, but it is obvious enough that the body and hence its internal environment can be invaded by physical objects and organisms from outside. It is affected by all kinds of physical, social and economic circumstances around it.

I may say that, as Governor-General, I run into environmental questions over and over again as I open or address a wide variety of conferences. In recent years the environmental issues have begun to affect most aspects of human life. For example, whenever engineers, miners, builders, architects, planners, real estate agents and many other groups on the physical and social side come together it is impossible nowadays for them to avoid discussing environmental matters.

The impact of the environment on disease has long been recognised in medicine and a wide variety of public health problems through history have been related to environmental factors. The sweeping effect on history of plague, pestilence and disease has been as much or more due to environmental factors as to the actual medical and scientific explanations of what has happened. Many branches of medicine, public, industrial, tropical, preventative and others, have for long been concerned with environmental considerations.

In the material which has been provided to me for the purposes of this address it has become clear that pathologists have a very direct interest, so far as cells and tissues of the body are concerned, with internal relationships in the organisation within the body of the bodily environment of particular cells and tissues. But part of the problem for the pathologist is also the way the whole body reacts to and interacts with what I have seen described as 'favourable and unfavourable factors in its environment'.

The specialty of pathology is facing up to a number of questions which current environmental discussion and controversy have raised. There has been undoubtedly a great increase in the general interest in both environmental conservation and the reaction between man and his environment.

I have been told that for this reason the Congress Committee has considered that it accords with present moves for environmental improvement to discuss and consider how external factors, chemical, physical, microbiological or even social, might adversely affect susceptible individuals.

In the past, pathology has done much to advance the frontiers of medical knowledge. Pathologists have played leading roles in such major areas of medicine as the control of infectious disease, particularly by antibiotics and immunisation. Today they are leading in the quest for the causes and cures for cancer. As a professional group they have much to be proud of in their past. Therefore it is interesting to note that one whole day of conference is being devoted to the 'future of pathology'.

This is a question of concern to many pathologists and health administrators today. The areas of most interest are not necessarily the scientific developments likely to occur, but the way in which pathology services will be organised – what will be the place of pathology in medicine and ultimately in our society? This is of importance not only to established pathologists, but also to aspiring pathologists and to governments and others organising medical resources.

Pathology is a branch of medicine that links the roles of clinical medicine and biological science. To a large extent the pathologist must be both a clinician and a scientist – a diagnostician and a researcher. Some may have a leaning towards the clinical areas; others, and particularly those in universities, may see themselves more as medical research scientists.

The role of the pathologist himself, both within his specialisation and within medicine in general, is being examined at the present time throughout the world. An examination, if you like, of the pathologist in relation to his environment. Such consideration has come about as a result of the rapid growth of the specialisation in pathology, the increasing array of sophisticated equipment which now identifies its practice, and the growing number of trained personnel including Ph.D. level scientists, technologists and technicians who are, to a large extent, relieving the pathologist of some of his former 'medical scientist' functions. It is worthy of note that this point is to be discussed at the Congress.

I should say that it is a very healthy sign that pathologists at a world congress are going to consider all these problems because, as they doubtless realize, persons in other specialties outside medicine are coming to recognise and refer to the direct connection between such environmental factors as, for example, poor housing, and I mention only one, and the pathological problems which can be associated with them. Such other specialties obviously need the detailed scientific help of the outward-looking pathologist who is willing not merely to detect and diagnose the nature of a disease but to track it outwards into the external world for its environmental causation when this is relevant.

One has only to look at any pollution control authority of the kind established in recent years by Governments to see that even the vocabulary they use must have medical and pathological implications. The very legislation widely enacted nowadays dealing with air pollution, water pollution and the pollution of noise must be related to medical problems as well as to merely cosmetic aspects of the environment itself, though I do not minimise those important aspects. Pollution is damaging not merely to the environment but also to people. It is well understood that the control of impurities and odours emitted into the air is necessary for many reasons, not the least of which is the achievement of long term goals of the World Health Organisation.

I have mentioned the language or vocabulary of the environmental institutions and movements. There is a commonly held view by most governmental authorities that they have a duty to prevent the entry of chemicals and materials into the environment, that they should control and regulate the disposal of solid, liquid, toxic, noxious, animal and radioactive wastes. Now, what do we mean by 'harmful' in this connection? What do we mean by 'toxic'? Radioactivity of course speaks for itself.

On environmental matters, architects, engineers and builders have in the past been accused of 'tunnel vision', that is to say of single-objective planning without due regard for the surrounding environment, both physical and social. This directs attention to the consequences on the environment of the unconcerned activities of those engaged in these professions and activities. It is, I believe, no longer fair to accuse these professions in this way. They have come a long way in recent years.

I should like to look, by way of analogy, at the medical profession and at pathology in this respect. It is clear enough from what I have said that many forms of pollution and other environmental factors can affect the body and its cells and tissues and that pathologists need to consider these matters. An important question is – should this drive medical people, especially pathologists, to try to protect the body and its cells and tissues from the environment by making difficult, indeed impossible, demands upon the environment for change? Should the body as far as possible be put into a cocoon?

The medical profession could do well to examine its own activities on this basis. The profession is concerned with the physical health of mankind and decisions in the public health field may be taken without sufficient recognition of the wider system of which human beings are a part, e.g.:

1. Drinking water and bathing water standards could be made too stringent when viewed in the wider perspective. To achieve these very stringent standards economic resources could be stretched in terms of provision of over designed treatment facilities restricting funds available for other activities which may affect the social environment of mankind.

2. Stringent public health requirements may alter the 'character' of a city. Small businesses which do not comply with regulations may be forced to close down where the real health hazard is not great.

In summary public health standards and regulations could be designed very drastically to minimise risk with respect to immediate physical health but in so doing could introduce problems in terms of environmental costs.

These are important questions of balance. Governmental environmental authorities generally stress not only what is technologically practicable but what is economically feasible, whilst accepting the principle that no one should have the uncontrolled right to contaminate the environment.

One of the enormously important environmental factors so far as man is concerned is mankind itself. By this I refer, of course, to the population problem – to the prospect, helped to realisation by medicine itself, of a huge increase in the numbers of humanity. In countries which are overpopulated this aspect of the environment has enormous medical and pathological implications.

All people including the medical profession must accept and understand certain facts about the earth, its limits of growth and the dangers of failing to accept the basic laws of the biosphere. We must recognise that we cannot conquer nature. We can only live within it and within its laws. The basic natural system is the biological life cycle and this requires us to remember two things. First, our economic systems must be adjusted to a necessary biological equilibrium and our medical systems, including the demands of pathology, must learn to adjust to the environmental limits.

It is one thing to demand that the environment be altered at enormous economic expense to provide a pathological heaven. It is another to understand that pathology must live in a finite world, on a finite planet with imposed social and biological limits on man's capacity to protect man from risks of disease. We must do our best whilst recognising that we fall short of being gods.

You are here looking at environmental problems as affecting the cells and tissues of the human body. I am not an expert in biology but even those of us who today go no further than simple popular biology have been taught, mainly by environmentalists, about ecosystems, namely systems in which a community of organisms interact with one another and with their physical environment. An ecosystem, we are told, includes everything, living and non-living in a defined area. Living in a habitat most living things, from the smallest microbe, are to some extent dependent on other living organisms – in a complex web of life. There is a dramatic interdependence which is an important feature of all ecosystems and affects all living species and organisms.

Normally we hear about ecology and ecosystems and the habitat when the wider questions of the environment are being discussed – namely the impact and often the adverse effect of man on his environment. But I should imagine that the same questions arise, though perhaps in smaller ecosystems, when we are considering the impact of his environment on man.

I have mentioned the problems of overpopulation as part of the environment of man with serious medical implications in many parts of the world. Food shortages and near starvation is often associated with this problem. Also connected with all of this is underdevelopment. Big political, economic and social problems are today being debated in international councils. The language of these debates and of environmentalists is often overdramatic but perhaps we need to have people using strong language to awaken us. They tell us that as populations explode, as habitats are destroyed the species and ecosystems with which we have journeyed through a thousand millenia are fast disappearing. Is this true? If it is even partly true, what are the consequences in the long term for pathology?

Of course many pathological issues must arise, in our man-made environment, in human settlements – villages, towns and cities. The broad aim of mankind, pursued through the ages by conflict and co-operation, has been to ensure the essentials of health, shelter, food, work and education and hence a quality of life worth having. All of these are interconnected and all, I should imagine, can in one way or another affect human pathology. What is now being argued by some is that what is now involved is the question, not of the continued provision of these things, but of man's very survival.

There are a number of special areas of environmental concern which can only be mentioned rather than discussed, and then only as examples. Take the consequences of the use of pesticides and related compounds, pollution by heavy metals such as lead and mercury, radiation, other sources including chemical sources of mutations and the epidemiological environment. I am told that we do not completely understand the behaviour of viruses but we do know that the development of highly lethal strains of human viruses and the invasion of humanity by extremely dangerous strains of animal viruses are possible. We also know that crowding increases the chances for development of a virus epidemic.

It seems to me that environmental health and environmental management are related. Some diseases whether water-borne or transmitted by insect vectors arise from man's engineering and mechanical skills. The preservation of the health of the community requires a multidisciplinary approach and problems of environmental health often require an engineering or technological solution.

In our scientific age it is impossible to avoid the conclusion that whatever adverse effects there have been from the past use of applied science and technology the continued resort to science and technology will be an essential element in handling problems of environmental health. Perhaps, like others who have tried to say a few words about this huge subject, I may be permitted in this company to conclude with a quotation from Sir Macfarlane Burnet's book, *Dominant Mammal: The Biology of Human Destiny:*

> A viable and humanly tolerable world – a stable human ecosystem for the earth – is conceptually, ecologically and socially possible, but it will not be reached unless men and women of vision, purpose and intelligence can devise ways of controlling, modifying and redirecting those patterns of behaviour that were consolidated in the course of human evolution and which have brought us to the brink of chaos.

1: What keeps tissues normal?

Nucleus, cytoplasm and their interactions

L. Goldstein

*Department of Molecular, Cellular and Developmental Biology,
University of Colorado, Boulder, Colo., U.S.A.*

That the nucleus and cytoplasm must interact for effective cell function can be demonstrated in numerous ways but none are as dramatic as that which shows neither compartment can survive in the absence of the other. Under the best of circumstances a nucleus removed from an animal cell can survive for only a matter of minutes, whereas the cytoplasm – which does somewhat better – can function without a nucleus for at most a few days. Knowledge of this kind of mutual interdependence tells us little, however, of the nature of the interactions between nucleus and cytoplasm; we still want to know what the interacting mechanisms are.

Some relatively simple things we know already. The cytoplasm, aside from acting as a protector from the harshness of the extracellular environment, provides the nucleus with such things as sources of energy, precursors of RNA and DNA synthesis, protein components of chromosomes and other nuclear structures, etc. In fact, since RNA and DNA synthesis is the only metabolic function that we can confidently assign to nuclei generally, conceivably all other components of most nuclei may be furnished by the cytoplasm. For materials travelling in the reverse direction we know with certainty only that the nucleus provides the cytoplasm with nucleic acid components of the translational machinery (i.e. the 28S, 18S and 5S RNAs of ribosomes, the amino acid transfer RNAs, and the multiplicity of messenger RNAs that serve as templates for protein synthesis). Conceivably, the nucleus provides the cytoplasm with some other kinds of RNAs having more specialized functions (Ro-Choi and Busch, 1974; Moscona et al., 1970; Bester et al., 1975), some of which may be important for subtle nucleocytoplasmic interactions, but beyond that there may be nothing furnished the cytoplasm by the nucleus.

Numerous other facets of nucleocytoplasmic interactions currently attract most attention, probably because they are more mysterious and seem to be concerned with regulatory functions. There are four research areas of particular interest: (1) cytoplasmic influences on specific gene expression; (2) cytoplasmic involvement in developmental processes; (3) interactions between cytoplasmic organelles and nucleus; and (4) nucleocytoplasmic interactions in certain pathological states.

Cytoplasmic influences on specific gene expression

This subject probably is basic to understanding most other aspects of nucleocytoplasmic interactions, which in turn are some of the more important problems of interest to contemporary experimental biologists. Although several model systems concerned with the control of gene expression have been studied for a number of years, we remain – by the standards of the accomplishments of bacterial cell investigators – largely ignorant of the fundamental mechanisms at work.

Probably the first model system that unambiguously showed the cytoplasm to be responsible for specifying which genes in a cell are expressed came from the work of Beale (1954) on the inheritance of surface antigens in the single-celled organism, Paramecium. Beale demonstrated that the particular surface antigen produced (which at any one time is limited to only one of a whole spectrum of gene-specified antigens) is determined by the cytoplasm into which the genes are introduced (as the result of transferral of a nucleus from one cell to another during sexual conjugation). What determines the state of the cytoplasm is the state of the extracellular environment. No great advances have been made since Beale's original work, so that we still do not know what it is about the cytoplasm that turns certain genes on and others off (but cf. Finger, 1975).

Although the next model system might more appropriately be included in the section on developmental processes following, I include it here because it deals with the effects on specific gene activity. Gurdon (1973) and his colleagues have performed a variety of nuclear transplantations between frog cells at various development stages from oogenesis to tadpoles and adults. As a result they have demonstrated that the specific kinds of RNAs, whether transfer RNAs, ribosomal RNAs, or heterogeneous nuclear RNAs (each of which is specified by different gene classes), that are made at a particular stage of development are determined by the kind of cytoplasm into which a nucleus of any differentiated cell is placed. In related kinds of experiments they showed that whether or not nuclear DNA is replicated is also determined by the nature of the recipient cytoplasm.

Hormone action often is manifested by altered expression of particular genes in the target organ cells. In the well-studied case of the mammalian uterus response to estrogen, the response to hormone administration has been shown to be an activation of the production of certain RNAs associated with the growth and proliferation of uterine cells (O'Malley and Means, 1974). We probably know more about the molecular events associated with the control of gene expression in this model system than in any other nucleated cells; in barest outlines, the following are the events as we currently understand them. Present in the cytoplasm are protein hormone receptors that are multimeric polypeptide complexes designated 8S. These specifically combine with estradiol when a sufficiently high hormone titer is reached, following which the 8S receptor is converted to a smaller, 5S-hormone complex. Whereas the 8S complex is unable to enter the nucleus, the 5S-hormone complex has a particular affinity for the nucleus and accumulates there. What follows in the nucleus is unclear but it appears that hormone is somehow able to associate with the chromatin – presumably with specific genetic loci, but that has not been demonstrated. This new association ostensibly is responsible for the transcription of genes heretofore inactive, resulting in the production of new mRNAs to be translated in the cytoplasm. In the context of our subject then, we can say that the cytoplasm influences specific gene function by responding to specific environmental stimuli. Obviously, if the 8S receptor complex were not present in the cytoplasm, as is the case in non-target tissues, there would be no genetic response.

An entirely different approach to the study of gene expression employs the production of cell hybrids, usually by fusing cells that show differing phenotypes and/or genotypes. (Most frequently cells are caused to fuse by administration of inactivated Sendai virus (Sidebottom, 1974).) In a pioneering series of studies Harris and his associates (reviewed by Sidebottom, 1974) carried out fusions between cultured mammalian cells (e.g. HeLa), which are actively engaged in DNA and RNA synthesis, and chick erythrocytes, which neither transcribe nor replicate their DNA; the nuclei of chick erythrocytes are genetically inert. As a result of such a fusion the two nuclei share the same cytoplasm, which for all practical purposes is almost entirely of mammalian origin. In such a 'hybrid' the chick nucleus is reactivated and resumes transcriptive and replicative activity. In other words, the mammalian cytoplasm has the same effect on the chick nucleus as it does on the mammalian nucleus, even though the nucleus and cytoplasm come from different taxonomic classes. Moreover, it is important to note that new protein products specified by chick genes are produced as a result of hybrid formation, i.e. not only are chick genes transcribed but the transcripts also are translated in mammalian cytoplasm. These experiments present some difficulty in pinpointing where the activating influence is located, since both the nucleus and cytoplasm of the activating partner are present. (A similar difficulty is encountered in analyzing the characteristics of the hybrid cells to be mentioned below.) Recently, Ege et al. (1975) showed that some reactivation of a chick nucleus can occur following fusion to enucleate mouse fibroblasts but, unfortunately, this 'hybrid' dies before full reactivation is achieved.

Many other kinds of cell fusions, which ultimately may prove to be more useful for understanding how gene expression is controlled under normal in vivo conditions, have been performed. In ideal experiments fusions between two kinds of cells displaying one or a few differences in specific gene expression are effected and the consequences noted (Davis and Adelberg, 1973). For example, when cells of two cultured rat liver cell lines – HTC, which produces tyrosine aminotransferase (TAT) in response to steroid inducers, and BRL-62, which cannot produce the enzyme under any circumstances – are fused, the resultant hybrids are unable to synthesize TAT in response to appropriate stimuli (Thompson and Gelehrter, 1971). It is important to note that, since the two cell lines derive from rats of the same inbred strain, they probably have close to identical genotypes. If so, it follows that the different phenotypes reflect developmental differentiations that are probably due to cytoplasmic differences. Analysis of various factors that might be responsible for the phenotype of the hybrid suggests that most likely the hybrid displays no TAT activity because the BRL-62 partner contributes a factor that represses the expression of the relevant gene in the HTC nucleus. My guess is that the factor will be located in the cytoplasm (and is, in some sense of the word, 'self-perpetuating'). To establish that (as well as the nature of the precise effectors in other kinds of fusions) will require fusions of the nucleus of one cell line with the cytoplasm of the other – an accomplishment now shown to be possible (Veomett et al., 1974).

Cytoplasmic influences in development

Differential gene expression and its control is the essence of much of embryonic development. This section is placed here (rather than being incorporated into the preceding one) because we remain fairly ignorant of the specific molecular events of development and yet certain general phenomena are important for our comprehension of the problem. Although many examples of cytoplasmic influences on developmental processes are known, only three will be cited as illustrative of the kind of phenomena considered worthy of study.

A casual reading of some relevant current literature would not lead one to the realization that the old-time biologists were more than a little knowledgeable about these matters, yet there is no doubt that at the turn of the century embryologists were fully aware that the cytoplasm played a central role in development –despite the fact that almost all the information for ontogeny resides in the nucleus. Thus, they were able to draw quite precise 'fate maps' of a great variety of mosaic eggs, in which the regions of an uncleaved egg (possessor of only one nucleus) were accurately delineated with respect to the specific tissue that would ultimately arise from each region (Willier et al., 1955). Obviously, this delineation must reside in the cytoplasm.

Of more recent vintage are the classic nuclear transplantation experiments of Gurdon (1974). Gurdon and his colleagues have shown that amphibian nuclei (and by extension nuclei of all multicellular organisms) of essentially all developmental stages and tissues tested, including e.g. larval intestine and adult skin, retain the capacity to support full normal development when transplanted to enucleate eggs. This means, of course, that no permanent changes occur in these nuclei as the cells in which they reside become more and more specialized in the course of development. Moreover, this also means that, by transferring a nucleus from one kind of cytoplasm to another, the entire spectrum of genes being expressed can be altered. One can reasonably generalize from this observation that the cytoplasm (or the environment acting upon the cytoplasm, as in the case of hormone actions mentioned above) is what is primarily responsible for the control of gene expression during much of development.

A more subtle developmental process than the aforementioned ones is called 'determination'. A cell is considered to be determined when it is irreversibly committed to a particular differentiated state but displays none of the characteristics of that state nor any other change from its pre-determined state, at which time its differentiation potential was presumably much more broad. Garcia-Bellido and Merriam (1971) have demonstrated for Drosophila development that alteration (by X-irradiation) of the genetic make-up of a particular larval or pupal cell may affect the nature of the specific genes in the cell but will not alter which genes are destined to be expressed – if the alteration occurs after the onset of determination but prior to the beginning of the specific cell differentiation. In other words, once determination has occurred it persists (apparently as a cytoplasmic state) regardless of what is done to the nucleus. In fact, the determined cell with the altered nucleus can proceed through a few cell divisions before the specific differentiation is manifested. We can conclude, therefore, that the determined state is one which can be replicated in the cytoplasm, or at least is heritable through the cytoplasm.

Interactions between nucleus and cytoplasmic organelles

In the course of what we consider 'typical' cell growth and reproduction everything in the cell must double: chromosomes, ribosomes, mitochondria, etc. Obviously, this requires extremely fine-tuned coordination of a host of meta-bolic activities to ensure that no significant imbalance in the production of any organelle occurs; in fact, most imbalances reflect pathological conditions. Of unique interest is the coordination between the reproduction of so-called semi-autonomous organelles, i.e. mitochondria and chloroplasts, and that of the rest of the cell. This interest arises because these semi-autonomous organelles possess their own chromosomes, which replicate independently of the nuclear chromosomes, yet just one net doubling of each kind of genome occurs per cell generation. If the organelle were to replicate less than once per cell generation, the organelles would eventually be lost; if the organelle were to replicate more than once per cell generation, the organelles would eventually overwhelm the cell. Hence, the obvious need for close integration of the activities of the two kinds of cellular genomes.

A brief look at chromosome replication provides some notion of the dimen-sions of the problem. Although much needs to be learned about the regulation of nuclear DNA replication, we are fairly certain that cytoplasmic factors must play a significant role in the precise initiation of DNA synthesis at a specific point in the cell cycle and that cytoplasmic factors may play a part in the termi-nation of DNA synthesis following an exact doubling of chromosomal DNA. We know that in most cells the aforementioned cytoplasmic factors play no role in organellar DNA synthesis for the simple reason that the latter process occurs at times quite different from that in the nucleus. Moreover, while nuclear DNA synthesis usually requires several hours to be complete, the small amount of organellar DNA can be replicated in a few minutes, yet, because there are many organelles per cell and their replication is not synchronous, organellar DNA synthesis often occurs through most of the cell cycle. Nevertheless, there is but one doubling of total organellar DNA per cell cycle. We obviously are confront-ed with processes that are independently regulated yet somehow closely coord-inated. How is that achieved?

It is not difficult to imagine how that is achieved, although we do not in fact know how it is done. Although organelles are composed of many different kinds of proteins and RNAs, the organelle chromosomes (especially of mitochondria) possess far too little DNA to code for all the macromolecules of the organelles. It follows then that much of the material must be specified by the nucleus and that the availability of nuclear-coded organellar products may serve to coordinate the two kinds of reproduction. Numerous nucleus-specified organellar proteins are now known (Mahler, 1973) which might serve the coordinating function but we have few clues as to how they might do so. Some of these clues are the following.

The number of organelles in a cell apparently is related to the amount of chromatin in the nucleus. In yeast, the amount of mitochondrial DNA is proportional to the amount of nuclear DNA, which varies according to the particular strain of yeast (Mahler, 1973). Studies of a great variety of plants similarly have shown a close correlation between the nuclear ploidy or an organism and the number of chloroplasts per cell (Butterfass, 1973). This relation is true even when environmental (rather than genetic) factors cause alterations in nuclear DNA content.

Certain organellar enzyme complexes are composed of some polypeptides coded for by the nuclear genome and some by the organellar genome. These obviously provide a favorable locus for coordination. One such complex is the cytochrome oxidase system of Neurospora (Lansman et al., 1974). In the presence of cycloheximide, which inhibits protein synthesis directed by the nucleus but not that of the organelle, the cytochrome oxidase subunits coded by mitochondrial DNA are produced but not integrated into the enzyme complex. They may be integrated following the removal of cycloheximide. However, the longer the cycloheximide treatment, the more unstable are the mitochondrial-coded subunits and, thus, they are less and less able to be integrated. Therefore, if the important enzyme complex cytochrome oxidase is essential for mitochondrial growth, we can imagine that the amount of cytochrome oxidase subunit mRNA being transcribed in the nucleus could serve to limit the organellar growth rate. Similar kinds of results have been obtained using genetic mutants (rather than inhibitors) to block the production of one kind of mitochondrial respiratory complex subunit or another (Ebner et al., 1973a, b).

Probably the best understood and most interesting system coded for by both genomes is the so-called Fraction I protein of chloroplasts (Smith, 1975). This complex carries the catalytic function of ribulose-1,5-diphosphate carboxylase, the enzyme activity responsible for photosynthetic carbon fixation. This enzyme complex, which is the major protein of chloroplasts and has a molecular weight of ca. 5.25×10^5 daltons, probably consists of 8 identical subunits of ca. 55,000 daltons and 8-10 identical small subunits of ca. 15,000 daltons. Several invest-igators (Sakano et al., 1974; Gray and Kekwick, 1973) have shown by genetic analysis, in vitro protein synthesis by chloroplasts, and inhibitor experiments that the large subunit is specified by chloroplast genes and the small subunit by nuclear genes. The striking recent finding in this system is that when the produc-tion of the small subunit is inhibited, the production (not merely the accumula-tion) of the large subunit by chloroplasts is blocked. Thus, one can imagine that the small subunit itself directly regulates chloroplast synthesis of the large sub-unit.

Finally, we can note that regulation by organelles of the nuclear activity may also occur. In the alga Chlamydomonas inhibition of chloroplast transcription or translation will block nuclear DNA synthesis long before there is any effect on organelle DNA synthesis (Blamire et al., 1974).

Interactions of nucleus and cytoplasm in certain pathological states

Knowledge of nuclear and cytoplasmic interactions in cells under particular pathological conditions will not necessarily lead to a full understanding of the responsible mechanisms but such an understanding should at least help de-lineate important features that deserve further study.

There are two conditions, cancer and ageing, that seem particularly well suited for investigations of nucleocytoplasmic interactions and recent develop-ments have created an especially optimistic climate for progress. Of great poten-tial value is the achievement by Veomett et al. (1974) of a method for 'reconsti-tuting' cultured mammalian cells by recombining the nucleus of one cell with the cytoplasm of another. This method can be utilized to create a cell composed of a nucleus from a cancer cell and the cytoplasm of a non-cancer cell, or vice versa, and noting the characteristics of such a 'hybrid'. Similar experiments can, of course, be performed with senescent and non-senescent cells. Results from such experiments have not yet been reported but they are eagerly awaited.

Molecules involved in interactions between cytoplasm and nucleus

In only a few instances, such as the action of estrogens on target cells, do we have any clues as to the molecular mechanisms by which interactions between cyto-plasm and nucleus are effected. One approach to discovering those mechanisms is to identify the molecules that necessarily effect the interactions and to describe how they work. Likely candidates for these roles are a variety of RNA and protein molecules that migrate non-randomly between cytoplasm and nucleus. Studies on such molecules have been reviewed recently (Goldstein, 1974).

References

Beale, G. H. (1954): *The Genetics of Paramecium aurelia.* Cambridge University Press, Cambridge.

Bester, A. J., Kennedy, D. S. and Heywood, S. M. (1975): *Proc. nat. Acad. Sci. (Wash.), 72,* 1523.

Blamire, J., Flechtner, V. R. and Sager, R. (1974): *Proc. nat. Acad. Sci. (Wash.), 71,* 2867.

Butterfass, T. (1973): *Protoplasma (Wien), 76,* 167.

Davis, F. M. and Adelberg, E. A. (1973): *Bact. Rev., 37,* 197.

Ebner, E., Mason, T. L. and Schatz, G. (1973 b): *J. biol. Chem., 248,* 5369.

Ebner, E., Mennucci, L. and Schatz, G. (1973 a): *J. biol. Chem., 248,* 5360.

Ege, T., Zeuthen, J. and Ringertz, N. R. (1975): *Somat. Cell Genet., 1,* 65.

Finger, I. (1975): In: *Paramecium: A Current Survey,* p. 131. Editor: W. J. Van Wagtendonk. Elsevier Publishing Co., Amsterdam.

Garcia-Bellido, A. and Merriam, J. R. (1971): *Proc. nat. Acad. Sci. (Wash.), 68,* 2222.

Goldstein, L. (1974): In: *The Cell Nucleus, Vol. I,* p. 387. Editor: H. Busch. Academic Press, New York.

Gray, J. C. and Kekwick, R. G. O. (1973): *FEBS Letters, 38,* 67.

Gurdon, J. B. (1973): *Brit. med. Bull., 29,* 259.

Gurdon, J. B. (1974): In: *The Cell Nucleus, Vol. I,* p. 471. Editor: H. Busch. Academic Press, New York.

Lansman, R. A., Rowe, M. J. and Woodward, D. O. (1974): *Europ. J. Biochem., 41,* 15.

Mahler, H. R. (1973): In: *Molecular Cytogenetics,* p. 181. Editors: B. A. Hamkalo and J. Papaconstantinou. Plenum Press, New York.

Moscona, A. A., Moscona, M. and Jones, R. E. (1970): *Biochem. biophys. Res. Commun., 39,* 943.

O'Malley, B. W. and Means, A. R. (1974): In: *The Cell Nucleus, Vol. III,* p. 379. Editor: H. Busch. Academic Press, New York.

Ro-Choi, T. S. and Busch, H. (1974): In: *The Cell Nucleus, Vol. III,* p. 152. Editor: H. Busch. Academic Press, New York.

Sakano, K., Kung, S. D. and Wildman, S. G. (1974): *Molec. gen. Genet., 130,* 91.

Sidebottom, E. (1974): In: *The Cell Nucleus, Vol. I,* p. 439. Editor: H. Busch. Academic Press, New York.

Smith, H. (1975): *Nature (Lond.), 254,* 13.

Thompson, E. B. and Gelehrter, T. D. (1971): *Proc. nat. Acad. Sci. (Wash.), 68,* 2589.

Veomett, G., Prescott, D. M., Shay, J. and Porter, K. R. (1974): *Proc. nat. Acad. Sci. (Wash.), 71,* 1999.

Willier, B. H., Weiss, P. A. and Hamburger, V. (Ed.) (1955): *Analysis of Development.* W. B. Saunders Co., Philadelphia.

Lineages, quantal cell cycles and cell diversification*

H. Holtzer and S. Holtzer

Department of Anatomy, School of Medicine,
University of Pennsylvania, Philadelphia, Pa., U.S.A.

Much work over the past two decades has attempted to demonstrate a primary role for exogenous molecules and cell-cell interactions in diversifying 'undifferentiated' or 'multipotential' cells (Fleischmajer and Billingham, 1968; Rutter et al., 1973; Slavkin and Greulich, 1975). In our opinion this vast literature in fact demonstrates that exogenous molecules merely permit already diversified cells to express metabolic options that otherwise might remain unexpressed. Cell-cell interactions, nerve growth factor (Levi-Montalcini, 1974), colony-stimulating factors (Metcalf, 1974; Till et al., 1974) etc. at most function as hormones (Holtzer, 1968; Holtzer et al., 1972). They cue already diversified target cells that have been differentiated by earlier endogenous events. Hydrocortisone, for example, induces three very different metabolic reactions in chondroblasts, liver cells and oocytes respectively. Clearly, even before being exposed to the hormone the chondroblast, the liver cell, or the oocyte was primed to respond, each

---

* This work was supported by NIH grants CA-18194, GM-20138, and HL15835 to the Pennsylvania Muscle Institute, and by grants from the Muscular Dystrophy Association and the National Science Foundation.

in its unique way, by prior diversifying events. Changes in a cell's microenvironment cannot be a primary 'cause' of cell diversification any more than a hormone can 'cause' the phenotype of its target cell. Though exogenous molecules may be required for the expression of a particular differentiated state, or influence a particular 'binary decision' (Abbott et al., 1974; Dienstman and Holtzer, 1975), in general they must be of secondary importance regarding the basic mechanisms of cell diversification.

Recently we have reviewed the old idea that lineages are central to cell diversification (Dienstman and Holtzer, 1975; Holtzer et al., 1975e). A scheme which postulates the passage of cells through an obligatory sequence of compartments within a lineage is incompatible with any scheme based on the diversification of virginal, undifferentiated cells by means of alterations in the cell's microenvironment. The concept of lineage excludes the existence of undifferentiated cells. The concept of lineage requires, however, a mechanism that promotes transit of cells through successive compartments within the lineage. It must also account for the way in which cells within one compartment, endowed with one set of circumscribed metabolic options, can yield daughter cells with predictably different metabolic options. We have proposed accordingly that transition from one compartment to the next requires reprogramming of the genome, and that this type of reprogramming – in contrast to changes induced by hormone like agents – requires DNA synthesis and passage through a 'quantal cell cycle'. By definition, a quantal cell cycle is one that allows a region of the genome that was not available for transcription in the mother cell to become available for transcription in the daughter cell (Holtzer et al., 1972; Dienstman and Holtzer, 1975; Holtzer et al., 1975e). Quantal cell cycles diversify by 'moving' cells from one compartment in the lineage into the next. This type of cell cycle differs from the more commonly studied cell cycle, the proliferative cell cycle, in which the daughter's options for transcription do not differ from those of the mother. Proliferative cell cycles increase the numbers of cells within a compartment. The mosaic type of developmental system is characterized by a succession of quantal cell cycles with no intervening proliferative cell cycles, whereas regulative systems permit variable numbers of proliferative cycles between the fixed number of quantal cell cycles.

Erythrogenesis

During erythrogenesis there may be no more than 5 quantal cell cycles separating the zygote from the 1st generation erythroblast (Holtzer et al., 1972; Holtzer et al., 1975e; Weintraub, 1975). Here we will focus on that quantal cell cycle effecting transit from the erythrogenic hematocytoblast compartment.

The primitive line of chick erythroblasts develop as a relatively homogenous cohort of cells and the Hb can be measured microspectrophotometrically in individual cells (Weintraub et al., 1971; Campbell et al., 1971). The erythrogenic hematocytoblasts do not synthesize Hb. However, by the time their daughter cells, the 1st generation erythroblasts, are only a few hours old they synthesize detectable quantities of Hb. Experiments based on uptake of ^{3}H-TdR demonstrated that a single erythrogenic hematocytoblast divides symmetrically, yielding two 1st generation erythroblasts (Campbell et al., 1971; Hagopian et al., 1972). These 1st generation erythroblasts serve as progenitors for six subsequent generations of erythroblasts. Each class of erythroblasts synthesizes characteristic amounts of Hb and displays characteristic cytologies and characteristic G1, S and G2 periods. The hematocytoblast and at least two different classes of erythroblasts coexist in the same circulation. This finding means that microenvironmental influences alone cannot influence the cell divisions that separate one class of erythroblast from another, nor induce that cell division which separates erythrogenic hematocytoblast from 1st generation erythroblast. These and other observations (Holtzer et al., 1975e; Weintraub, 1975) have led us to conclude that the hematocytoblast is endogenously programmed in such a way that its daughter erythroblasts serve as progenitors for only six generations, or 128 Hb-producing cells. This limited potential for replication of 1st generation erythroblasts is also displayed by other Hb-producing cells. Once normal erythrogenic cells or Friend leukemic cells induced with dimethyl sulfoxide initiate the synthesis of Hb, they function under stringent restraints with regard to DNA synthesis. There are no tumors in which each neoplastic cell synthesizes large quantities of Hb. Cells synthesizing significant quantities of Hb do not have the option to yield the large progeny that characterize 'stem' cells earlier in the lineage. A 1st generation erythroblast yields 128 descendants, whereas a 5th generation erythroblast yields two postmitotic daughters.

Current evidence favors the notion that a given erythrogenic hematocytoblast divides symmetrically, yielding two 1st generation erythroblasts. This means that, with respect to the broader hematopoietic lineages, the erythrogenic hematocytoblast must be past the binary decision point (Abbott et al., 1974; Dienstman and Holtzer, 1975; Holtzer et al., 1975e) where a given stem cell had the option to divide asymmetrically and establish white and red blood cell lineages respectively.

With regard to Hb synthesis there are significant differences between the erythrogenic hematocytoblasts and the erythroblasts in response to BudR and to the DNA inhibitors, cytarabine and FudR (Weintraub et al., 1972). Incorporation of BudR into the DNA of replicating erythroblasts does not block these cells from continuing to synthesize Hb. In contrast, incorporation of BudR into the DNA of replicating erythrogenic hematocytoblasts blocks the initiation of Hb synthesis in cells that otherwise would have begun to synthesize this molecule (Campbell et al., 1974). Blocking DNA synthesis with either cytarabine or FudR does not block any class of erythroblast from continuing to synthesize Hb. Indeed cytarabine-blocked 3rd generation erythroblasts continue to make Hb until their content exceeds that of 4th generation erythroblasts. These blocked cells enlarge greatly and eventually lyse. In contrast, cytarabine-treated hematocytoblasts do not initiate the synthesis of Hb. If embryos rich in erythrogenic hematocytoblasts are blocked from synthesizing DNA before erythroblasts have emerged, they never synthesize Hb. Taken together, these experiments show that movement from the penultimate compartment into the erythroblast compartment is not simply dependent upon 'maturation' of the erythrogenic hematocytoblast. The hematocytoblast itself cannot become an erythroblast. Only if the erythrogenic hematocytoblast synthesizes DNA and completes its nuclear division will cells emerge that have the option to synthesize Hb. Work to be published elsewhere has demonstrated that the relationship between the absence of Hb in the hematocytoblasts and its presence in their daughter erythroblasts also extends to the appearance of spectrin and carbonic anhydrase.

To determine whether the failure of erythrogenic hematocytoblasts to synthesize Hb was due to a failure in transcription or translation, the following experiments were performed. ^{3}H-cDNA against adult Hb-mRNA was prepared using *E. coli* reverse transcriptase (Groudine et al., 1974). Hybridization experiments with this labelled probe revealed that if globin message was transcribed in the erythrogenic hematocytoblast it was less than 10^{-5} times that found in erythroblasts. From this we concluded that: (1) erythrogenic hematocytoblasts did not transcribe active or inactive globin messages, and (2) one consequence of the quantal cell cycle was to make the globin genes that were not available for transcription in the hematocytoblast available for transcription in their daughter erythroblasts. Needless to say it would be of interest to know whether BudR and the Friend leukemic virus act on the same 'master locus' and that it is this locus that is altered during passage through the quantal cell cycle which separates the hematocytoblast from the erythroblasts.

Myogenesis

Since the crucial role of quantal cell cycles during myogenesis has been reviewed recently (Dienstman and Holtzer, 1975; Holtzer et al., 1975e) only a brief account will be sketched here. If it is assumed that the same mesenchyme cell

(Ms cell) is the common progenitor to the myogenic, chondrogenic, and fibrogenic lineages, then at a minimum three quantal cell cycles separate the Ms cell from the postmitotic myoblast. One quantal cell cycle separates the Ms cell from the PMbFb compartment and the PCbFb compartment. The PMbFb cell is a bipotential cell that yields a presumptive myoblast and/or definitive fibroblast, whereas the PCbFb cell is a bipotential cell that yields a chondroblast and/or fibroblast (Abbott et al., 1974; Dienstman and Holtzer, 1975; Holtzer et al., 1975e).

The abrupt switch in metabolic options which accompanies a quantal cell cycle is best documented by observing the changes in synthesis of the myosin heavy and light chains by presumptive myoblasts on the one hand and their daughter postmitotic myoblasts on the other. It has been known for years that replicating presumptive myoblasts do not bind labelled antibody against skeletal myosin, whereas their postmitotic daughters, the myoblasts, do (Holtzer et al., 1957; Okazaki and Holtzer, 1965). These old findings have recently been confirmed by collecting large numbers of mononucleated, postmitotic myoblasts with Cytochalasin-B and EGTA (Holtzer et al., 1975a, b).

By culturing replicating presumptive myoblasts, fibroblasts, chondroblasts and BudR-suppressed myogenic cells in ^{14}C-leucine, it can be shown that all of these kinds of cells synthesize a 200,000 myosin heavy chain. The myosins from these cells in dodecyl sulfate are indistinguishable from the myosins isolated from myoblasts, myotubes and mature muscle. Nevertheless, in Ouchterlony diffusion plates antibody against skeletal heavy chains does not even cross-react with the myosins from presumptive myoblasts or from non-myogenic cells. These findings confirm the suggestion (Holtzer et al., 1973) that the myosin heavy chain synthesized in the myoblast is the product of a different structural gene from that active in its mother, the replicating presumptive myoblast. These results are contrary to the many reports by Yaffe and co-workers (Yaffe, 1969; Yaffe and Dym, 1973) and by Strohman and co-workers (Paterson and Strohman, 1972; Przybyla and Strohman, 1974). Work in progress is designed to determine whether the myosin in replicating presumptive myoblasts is the product of the same structural gene active in such non-myogenic cells as fibroblasts, chondroblasts and nerve cells. If this should prove to be the case this myosin might be considered a 'constitutive' contractile protein.

Given current interest in contractile proteins in non-muscle cells, it is worth mentioning that the myosin molecules assembled into thick filaments in myoblasts are different from those that may be associated with (a) the outside of the plasma membrane (Willingham et al., 1974), or (2) the microfilaments subtending the plasma membrane (Weber and Groeschel-Stewart, 1974). Needless to say, the issue of polymorphism of a molecule such as myosin gives a new dimension to the problem of cell diversification (Holtzer, 1976).

Chi et al. (1975, 1976) have found comparable differences in the myosin light chains synthesized by myoblasts versus those synthesized by presumptive myoblasts and non-myogenic cells. Myoblasts synthesize the definitive light chains found in mature skeletal muscle. They have molecular weights of 25,000 and 18,000 respectively. Presumptive myoblasts and non-myogenic cells (e.g. fibroblasts, chondroblasts, nerve cells and BudR-suppressed myogenic cells) synthesize two light chains that are indistinguishable from one another in dodecyl sulfate gels; their molecular weights are 20,000 and 16,000. Again the issue is open as to whether these are 'constitutive' light chains common to all cells, whereas the definitive myoblasts synthesize their characteristic light chains only after passing through their terminal quantal cell cycle.

The mother of the postmitotic myoblast, the replicating presumptive myoblast, does not have the option to fuse to form myotubes (Dienstman and Holtzer, 1975; Okazaki and Holtzer, 1965; Holtzer et al., 1975c) or to initiate the synthesis of the definitive myosin heavy and light chains. These are the unique properties of postmitotic myoblasts. This transition between replicating presumptive myoblast and myoblast is not dependent upon collagen (Hauschka and Konigsberg, 1966; Konigsberg, 1972) or other mysterious factors in conditioned medium. Transition, however, is blocked by the incorporation of BudR into the DNA of the presumptive myoblast (Okazaki and Holtzer, 1965; Stockdale et al., 1964; Bischoff and Holtzer, 1969). BudR-suppressed myogenic cells do not withdraw from the cell cycle. Operationally the analog appears to promote proliferative cycles and thus preclude the quantal cell cycle required for transit into the myoblast compartment. In this regard BudR in the DNA of presumptive myoblasts mimics the effect of RSV on transformed myogenic cells (Holtzer et al., 1975d).

If presumptive myoblasts are treated with cytarabine or FudR they do not acquire the cell surface required for fusion nor do they initiate the synthesis of the definitive myosin heavy and light chains (Holtzer et al., 1973; Yeoh and Holtzer, 1976).

Clearly there are striking differences in the metabolic options open to the myoblast as compared to those available to their mother cells, the presumptive myoblast. Currently we are performing experiments based on the assumption that the differences between the two types of cells is due to activation of a 'master switch' that in turn makes available for transcription those myosin genes that are uniquely active in myoblast; it is assumed that the genes for such myosins are not available for transcription in the mother presumptive myoblast.

Summary

Much confusion in the literature could be avoided if the genetic regulation of a given cell's on-going metabolic activity was not confused with the regulatory mechanisms responsible for cell diversification. With this distinction in mind there is no reason to postulate different mechanisms between 'determination' and 'differentiation', or between regulative and mosaic systems. Fortunately there is a simple operational test for this distinction: if mother and daughter cells respond in a similar fashion to all exogenous molecules, then they are separated by a proliferative cell cycle and one is studying cell physiology. If there is a difference, then mother and daughter were separated by a quantal cell cycle and they have diversified.

It is obvious that the role of the quantal cell cycle in generating metabolic options in daughters that were not available in the mother cell is not synonymous with simply altering the synthetic activity of a given cell. The striking changes in response to exogenous influences in protozoan and metazoan cells without an intervening cell cycle, proliferative or quantal, are too well known to enlarge on here. What is being stressed is that there is one regulatory mechanism that (1) determines which of the available metabolic options a cell will use, and another that (2) determines which set of available options a cell will be endowed with. The former involves problems in cell physiology, the latter the unique problem of cell diversification. Much confusion and irrelevant semantics could be avoided by recognizing these two very different aspects of a given cell's metabolic behavior.

References

Abbott, J., Schiltz, J., Dienstman, S. and Holtzer, H. (1974): *Proc. nat. Acad. Sci. (Wash.), 71*, 1506.
Bischoff, R. and Holtzer, H. (1969): *J. Cell Biol., 41*, 188.
Campbell, G., Weintraub, H. and Holtzer, H. (1974): *J. Cell Physiol., 83*, 11.
Campbell, G., Weintraub, H., Mayall, B. and Holtzer, H. (1971): *J. Cell Biol., 50*, 669.
Chi, J., Fellini, S. and Holtzer, H. (1976): *Proc. nat. Acad. Sci. (Wash.)*, in press.
Chi, J., Rubinstein, N., Shrahs, K. and Holtzer, H. (1975): *J. Cell Biol.*, in press.
Dienstman, S. and Holtzer, H. (1975): In: *Cell Cycle and Cell Differentiation*. Editors: Reinert and H. Holtzer. Springer-Verlag, Heidelberg.
Fleischmajer, R. and Billingham, R. (ed.) (1968): *Epithelial-Mesenchymal Interactions*. Williams and Wilkins, Baltimore.
Groudine, M., Holtzer, H., Scherrer, K. and Therwath, A. (1974): *Cell, 3*, 243.
Hagopian, H., Lippke, J. and Ingram, V. (1972): *J. Cell Biol., 54*, 98.
Hauschka, S. and Konigsberg, I. (1966): *Proc. nat. Acad. Sci., (Wash.), 55*, 119.

Holtzer, H. (1968): In: *Epithelial-Mesenchymal Interactions.* Editors: R. Fleischmajer and R. Billingham. Williams and Wilkins, Baltimore.

Holtzer, H. (1976): *Cold Spr. Harb. Symp. quant. Biol.,* in press.

Holtzer, H., Biehl, J., Yeoh, G., Maganathan, R. and Kaji, A. (1975d): *Proc. nat. Acad. Sci. (Wash.)* in press.

Holtzer, H., Croop, J., Dienstman, S., Ishikawa, H. and Somlyo, A. (1975a): *Proc. nat. Acad. Sci. (Wash.), 72,* 513.

Holtzer, H., Marshall, J. and Finck, H. (1957): *J. Cell Biol., 3,* 705.

Holtzer, H., Rubinstein, N., Dienstman, S., Chi, J., Biehl, J. and Somlyo, A. (1975c): *Biochimie, 56,* 1575.

Holtzer, H., Rubinstein, N., Fellini, S., Chi, J. and Okayama, M. (1975e): *Quart. Rev. Biophysics.,* November.

Holtzer, H., Sanger, J., Ishikawa, H. and Strahs, K. (1973): *Cold Spr. Harb. Symp. quant. Biol., 37,* 549.

Holtzer, H., Strahs, K., Biehl, J., Somlyo, A. and Ishikawa, H. (1975b): *Science, 188,* 943.

Holtzer, H., Weintraub, H. and Mayne, R. (1972): In: *Current Topics in Developmental Biology.* Editors: Moscona and Monroy. Academic Press, New York.

Konigsberg, I. (1972): In: *Chemistry and Molecular Biology of the Intercellular Matrix, 3,* 1779. Editor: E. Balazs. Academic Press, New York and London.

Levi-Montalcini, R. (1974): In: *Dynamics of Degeneration and Growth in Neurons.* Editors: K. Fuxe, L. Olson and Y. Zotterman. Pergamon Press, Oxford.

Metcalf, D. (1974): *Cold Spr. Harb. Symp. quant. Biol., 38,* 887.

Okazaki, K. and Holtzer, H. (1965): *J. Histochem. Cytochem., 13,* 726.

Paterson, B. and Strohman, R. (1972): *Develop. Biol., 29,* 112.

Przybyla, A. and Strohman, R. (1974): *Proc. nat. Acad. Sci. (Wash.), 71,* 662.

Rutter, W., Pictet, R. and Monis, P. (1973): *Ann. Rev. Biochem., 42,* 601.

Slavkin, H. and Greulich, R. (1975): *Extracellular Matrix Influences on Gene Expression.* Academic Press, New York.

Stockdale, F., Nameroff, M., Okazaki, K. and Holtzer, H. (1964): *Science, 146,* 533.

Till, J., Messner, H., Price, G., Aye, M. and McCulloch, E. (1974): *Cold Spr. Harb. Symp. quant. Biol., 38,* 907.

Weber, K. and Groeschel-Stewart, U. (1974): *Proc. nat. Acad. Sci. (Wash.), 71,* 4561.

Weintraub, H. (1975) In: *Cell Cycle and Cell Differentiation.* Editors: Reinert and H. Holtzer. Springer-Verlag, Heidelberg.

Weintraub, H., Campbell, G. and Holtzer, H. (1972): *J. molec. Biol., 70,* 337.

Weintraub, H., Campbell, G., Mayall, B. and Holtzer, H. (1971): *Cell Biol., 50,* 652.

Willingham, M., Ostlund, R. and Pastan, I. (1974): *Proc. nat. Acad. Sci. (Wash.), 71,* 4144.

Yaffe, D. (1969): *Curr. Top. Develop. Biol., 4,* 37.

Yaffe, D. and Dym, H. (1973): *Cold Spr. Harb. Symp. quant. Biol., 37,* 543.

Yeoh, G. and Holtzer, H. (1976): *Exp. Cell Res.,* in press.

Adaptation to environmental changes: The role of cell-renewal systems*

T. M. Fliedner, K. H. Steinbach and D. Hoelzer

*Department of Clinical Physiology, University of Ulm,
Federal Republic of Germany*

Cellular homeostasis remains one of the great enigmas of human and mammalian biology, although the existence of a multicellular organism and its survival in changing environments is impossible without it. The term 'cellular homeostasis' represents the efficient performance and tremendous productivity by which the body maintains a dynamic equilibrium between cell production and cell removal. The histological picture of a tissue – such as liver, skin or bone marrow – cannot reflect the astonishing forces that keep all these tissues in a steady state. The balance maintained within a tissue, the cooperation between organ systems, and the equilibrium between the body and its physical, chemical and biological environment largely depend on the intact mechanisms of cellular homeostasis, the structural basis of which lies in the 'cell-renewal systems' (Fig. 1).

The significance of cellular homeostasis in cell systems is brought home when we realize that we recognize each other from one meeting to the next although the essential elements of the surface of our body – the epidermal epithelium – has

* Supported by the European Atomic Energy Community (EURATOM) and the Deutsche Forschungsgemeinschaft.

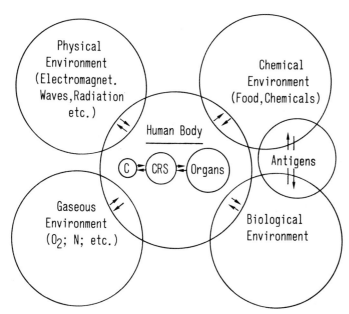

Fig. 1. Schematic representation of the relationship between the body and its environment and the role of cell-renewal systems. (C = cell; CRS = cell-renewal system.)

renewed itself many times in the interval. A physician expects to find an almost constant blood-cell count of erythrocytes, platelets and granulocytes from day to day in a healthy person. But it should be remembered that each day there is an entirely new granulocyte population, every 1-2 weeks a new platelet population and every quarter of a year a new erythrocyte population. It is also surprising to realize that our food is absorbed every week through a new layer of intestinal cells.

All this renewal activity normally occurs without our being aware of it. Nature has provided us, through cellular homeostasis, with an efficient demonstration that 'zero-growth' can occur simultaneously with continuous innovation, a lesson that should be recognized by many statesmen throughout the world today.

The purpose of this review is to describe the actual performance of cellular homeostasis by calculating the productivity of cell systems, to analyze their functional structure, and to examine present knowledge of the ways and means by which cell systems are adapted to special demands related to environmental conditions.

TABLE 1

Productivity of cell-renewal systems in the human body

Cell-renewal system	Production rate		
	cells/day (x 10^9)	cells/70 years (x 10^{14})	kg/70 years
Skin*	0.7	0.18	86
Mucosa of the gastro-intestinal tract*	56	14.31	6850
Lymphocytes	20	5.11	275**
Erythrocytes	200	51.10	460**
Granulocytes	120	30.66	5400**
Thrombocytes	150	38.33	40**

*   Croft and Cotton (1973).
** Based on a density of 1 g cm^{-3} and on the following cell volumes: lymphocytes 524 μm^3 (diameter 10 μm); erythrocytes 90 μm^3; granulocytes 1760 μm^3 (diameter 15 μm); thrombocytes 10 μm^3.

Productivity of cell-renewal systems

The tremendous achievements of cellular homeostasis can best be recognized by considering the extraordinary productivity of some human cell-renewal systems (Table 1).

The skin has an epithelial cell-renewal system that is essential for establishing and maintaining the exchange between the body and the environment. This vital barrier is also important for maintaining the 'milieu intérieur', as Claude Bernard (1878, quoted in Boylan, 1971) called it. It has been shown experimentally that at least 0.7×10^9 cells are formed every day, which represents a production of about 86 kg in 70 years.

The digestive tract has very active cell-renewal systems. Calculations show that these produce some 56×10^9 cells every day – equivalent to 6850 kg in 70 years. 90% of this production occurs in the small intestine, 9% in the colon and only 1% in the stomach.

The blood-cell forming tissues are also extraordinarily productive. A human being produces some 20×10^9 lymphocytes, 200×10^9 erythrocytes, 120×10^9 granulocytes and 150×10^9 platelets daily, equivalent to 275 kg, 460 kg, 5400 kg and 40 kg during a lifetime of 70 years.

These data indicate that cellular homeostasis is essential to the integrity of the body: if the body did not discard cells at the same rate as it produces them, it would grow to an impossible size. This actually occurs in neoplasia. Malignant growth is characterized by uncontrolled growth, in which cell production is not effectively balanced by cell loss. The cells accumulate without being removed and, thus, a tumor is produced. The rate at which a tumor grows depends on a number of factors, such as the growth fraction and the non-growth fraction, intratumoral cell deaths, and the environment. Studies on the extrapolation of tumor growth into the future on the basis of the observed growth pattern, e.g. in lung metastases, showed that, within a short time, the tumor would replace the body (National Cancer Institute, 1969). In one leukemic patient, we observed a progressive increase in leukemic blast cells in the blood. By repeated leukapheresis we were able to force the leukemic blood-cell concentration to level off when we had removed between 4.5 and 7.4×10^{11} leukocytes. In a period of 36 days about 4.78×10^{12} leukocytes were removed (98-99% blast cells), which is equivalent to at least 9 kg. From the number of cells removed, the net production rate of leukemic cells in this patient could be calculated as at least 1.2×10^{11} blast cells per day (Hoelzer et al., 1974). There is evidence that neoplasia is associated with impaired cell loss and cell destruction, but there are other conditions of hyperproduction with increased cell loss. The hemolytic anemias are an example of such increased cell system productivity (Nowicki et al., 1973). Other examples include: atrophic gastritis, with its particularly high rate of cell loss (3 times normal) (Croft et al., 1966), active celiac syndrome (4 times normal) (Croft et al., 1968; Trier and Browning, 1970) and psoriasis, in which the epithelial cell turnover and loss is 8 times normal (Croft et al., 1968a).

These abnormal states – tumors and hyperproductive diseases – clearly illustrate the significance of cellular homeostasis in cell-renewal systems. It seems essential to study the functional structure of these systems and their regulatory mechanisms.

Functional structure

The study of the various mammalian cell systems shows that their construction is similar in many respects in spite of the vast differences in their function and in the principles of their regulation.

The liver as an example of a latently resting cell system

The liver may be taken as an example of a cell system which in adult life – from the viewpoint of cell kinetics – is in a state of rest, though this rest is by no means static. No other system in the body is so dynamic. Greek mythology bears witness to this well-known fact: Prometheus was chained to a rock by Zeus as a

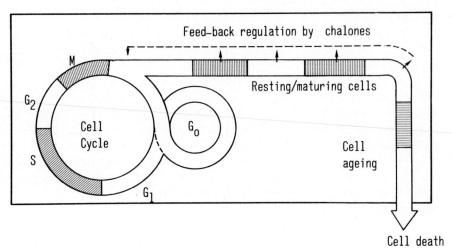

Fig. 2. Functional structure and regulation of latently resting cell systems: schematic representation of the liver system.

punishment. An eagle was sent every day to pick at his liver – symbolizing life itself – and the liver made up for the loss again and again by regeneration. In modern times, partial hepatectomy has been extensively used for studying the course and external and internal conditions of liver regeneration and the effects of nutrition, toxic substances, radiation, etc. From these studies (Grundmann, 1969; Maurer, 1973), an outline has emerged of the kinetic structure and regulation of the liver cell system – an example of a latently resting cell-renewal system (Fig. 2). According to this concept most of the parenchymal liver cells are normally at rest (in a 'G$_0$ state'). These cells can be recalled into the cellular cycle after appropriate stimulation, such as partial removal of liver tissue. They then enter the G$_1$ phase and undergo DNA synthesis, pass through the G$_2$ phase, and carry out mitosis. The newly formed cells can enter a new cell cycle or retire to a G$_0$ state. They can also 'mature' and are then incapable of responding again to a proliferative stimulus. Stöcker et al. (1972) have shown that more and more liver cells enter a G$_0$ state of 'no return' as the organism ages. However, if the liver of an old organism, with a reduced number of responsive G$_0$ cells, is triggered into proliferation by partial hepatectomy, the remaining 'responsive' G$_0$ cells then rebuild a new G$_0$ population with the same responsiveness as in a young organism. The mechanisms regulating the size of the normal liver cell system are being investigated in several laboratories. Proceeding from the theoretical growth model of Weiss and Kavanau (1957), the present theory of the mechanisms that keep the liver in a latent resting state holds that the major factors are inhibitory. The non-cycling cells produce an inhibitory factor (chalone) which prevents cells from entering the cell cycle and / or DNA synthesis (Verly et al., 1971; Stack-Dunne, 1973; Saetren, 1956). Partial hepatectomy either reduces the local concentration of an inhibitory factor or increases the level of a stimulatory factor, or both, until the tissue mass has regained its original size (Grundmann, 1969).

Epithelial cell-renewal systems

The epithelial cell-renewal systems of the skin and of the mucosa of the whole intestinal tract (from the lips to the anus) show additional features (Fig. 3). The skin contains a stem-cell pool as well as a pool of proliferative cells in the stratum basale. Some of the cells produced in this layer enter the pool of maturing cells in the stratum spinosum and stratum granulosum. Finally, the cells are discarded from the stratum corneum of the skin. According to Iversen (1969), this epidermal cell-renewal system is mainly regulated by a negative feed-back involving inhibitory factors (chalones). It is thought that the inhibitory factor is produced in cells of the stratum spinosum and stratum granulosum (Hondius Boldingh and Laurence, 1968; Oehlert, 1969), retained in the stratum corneum, and acts on the cells of the basal layer. A loss of differentiated cells from the system as well as an inhibition of cellular differentiation and a disruption of the skin would cause a local fall in the concentration of the inhibitor. Thus cells would be triggered to enter cellular division and differentiation (Iversen, 1969). In a recent series of experiments on mice, Rohrbach (1975) demonstrated that the concentration of one of the inhibitory factors is inversely proportional to the mitotic activity and that it is thus a mitosis-inhibiting factor. There is also evidence for a DNA synthesis-inhibiting factor; immediately before and during an increase in DNA synthesis there is a fall in the extractable inhibitory activity of the epidermis. From these studies it was concluded that there are inhibitory factors for both mitotic activity and DNA synthesis which are produced by differentiated epidermal cells during their maturation. If these cells are removed, the inhibitory activity disappears and cellular proliferation begins. Newly formed cell populations need a certain maturation time to produce a sufficient amount of inhibitory factors.

The functional structure of the mucous membranes of the intestinal tract is in principle similar to that of the skin (Fig. 3). In this review, the mouse small intestine will be used as an example. The cells of this system are produced continuously in Lieberkühn's crypts and pass through the neck of the crypts into the villi. There is a continuous flow of cells up the villi until they are discarded

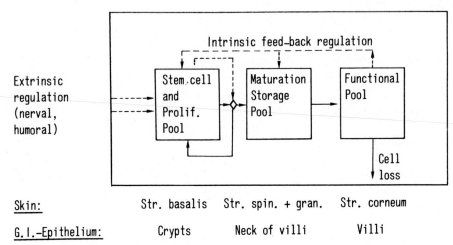

Fig. 3. Epithelial cell-renewal systems: schematic representation of the functional structure and regulation. Solid lines = cell flow. Broken lines = information flow.

into the intestinal lumen. As in the skin, cell production is quantitatively balanced by cell loss, and the rates of cell production, in man, are indicated in Table 1. The cell-renewal times in the intestinal epithelium have been estimated using tritiated thymidine. The villus transit time (transit through the functional pool, see Fig. 3) is the time between the first appearance of labeled cells at the base of the villi and the first labeled cells being shed from their tip. The villus transit time is 3-4 days in man, 2-3 days in rats and 1-2 days in mice (minimum estimates) (Bond et al., 1965). These figures should be treated with caution, since they vary from strain to strain in the same species and with age. The human studies were performed in cancer patients, which may have affected the time parameters. The cell-cycle times in the proliferative pool of the intestinal cell system in mice and rats were found to be 9-11 hours. It is interesting to note that the turnover of the cell system in the small intestine of mice was found to depend on the presence or absence of a microbial flora. Matsuzawa and Wilson (1965) found that the cell-cycle time of the intestinal cell system in germ-free mice was twice as long as in normal mice (38 vs. 19 hours), with a corresponding increase in the G_1, S, G_2 and M phases (Table 2).

The rate of movement along the villi was also found to differ in germ-free and normal mice. It takes 2.3 days for cells labeled with ^{3}H-TdR to reach the tip of the villus in normal animals, but 4.8 days in germ-free mice. It is noteworthy that in irradiated normal and germ-free mice the time for the loss of cells from the intestinal surface is directly related to this cell kinetic pattern. It takes 3-4 days

TABLE 2

Cell-cycle parameters in normal and germ-free mice

	Time (hr)	
	Normal	Germ-free
Generation	19	38
DNA	7.5	14.5
M phase	1	2
G₁ phase	9	18
G₂ phase	1.5	3

for normal mice to lose all villus cells after 3000 R of X-irradiation and 6-7 days in germ-free mice (Matsuzawa and Wilson, 1965). Accordingly, the diarrhea characteristic of the gastrointestinal syndrome after supralethal whole-body X-irradiation begins in normal mice after about 3 days and in germ-free mice after about 6 days (Bond et al., 1965).

These data are cited to indicate the cellular kinetics used as a basis for the system model in Figure 3. They also indicate that the renewal characteristics may be closely associated with, and actually dependent on, environmental conditions. In the particular case of the mouse, the renewal of the small intestine depends on the presence or absence of bacteria. This is a special case, probably due to the particular bile-acid metabolism of this species (Rankin et al., 1971), but emphasizes the fact that the homeostasis characteristic of a particular cell-renewal system may largely depend on environmental factors.

That epithelial cell-renewal systems of the intestinal mucosa can compensate for increased cell losses and still maintain an equilibrium between cell production and cell removal was shown in studies on rodents using continuous low-level X-irradiation. Lamerton and his associates performed extensive studies on the effects of continuous irradiation on the intestinal cell-renewal systems of rats and mice (Lesher et al., 1961, 1966). These indicate that the system can compensate by several mechanisms for increased cell loss due to exposure to X-rays in a dose of 50 rads per day. Initially (after 1 day), the movements of cells into or through mitosis are slowed and perhaps partly blocked in G₂. By 12 days there is evidence of a shortening of the generation cycle by 20%. However, this shortening of the generation time of the crypt cells is only temporary and it returns to normal values by 35 days in mice and 105 days in rats. The shortening of the crypt-cell generation time is thought to be a reaction by which the rodent compensates for the radiation-induced higher cell loss and maintains a normal mucosal cover on the villi. Morphologically, there seems to be a temporary extension of the zone of proliferation by movement of the proliferative boundary up the crypt and shortening of the villi.

A great deal is known about the adaptation of intestinal cell-renewal systems to environmental factors such as intestinal microbial flora or continuous low-level ionizing irradiation, but there is hardly any information about the mechanisms regulating the particular pattern of cellular homeostasis. Is it determined – like the skin – by inhibitory factors and hence controlled by the rate of loss of maturing cells? Does the loss of dividing-maturing cells trigger proliferation in neighboring cells? Are there also stimulatory factors triggering the cell cycle? Much more work must be done on the mucosal cell-renewal systems before the possibilities and limitations of the adaptation of these systems to environmental changes can be fully appreciated.

Hematopoietic cell-renewal systems

A third type of cell-renewal system occurs in hematopoietic tissue. These systems include important elements already described in relation to the liver and epithelial cell systems.

The hematopoietic cell systems are characterized by a functional pool of cells in the blood composed of erythrocytes, granulocytes, platelets, etc. (Fig. 4). The

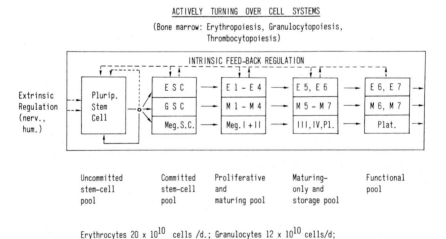

Erythrocytes 20 x 10^{10} cells /d.; Granulocytes 12 x 10^{10} cells/d;
Platelets 15 x 10^{10} cells/d.

Fig. 4. Schematic representation of hematopoietic cell-renewal systems and their intrinsic regulation. ESC = Erythropoietic stem cell; GSC = Granulopoietic stem cell; Meg.S.C. = Megakaryopoietic stem cell; Plat. = Platelets.

size of this pool is maintained by an influx of cells from the maturing and storage pool, quantitatively balancing the cell loss from the functional pool. There is a large pool of maturing granulocytes, but hardly any storage of non-dividing erythroblasts (orthochromatic normoblasts) or platelets. In these systems there is a pronounced dividing-maturing pool of cells where erythrocytic and granulo-cytic precursors undergo a series of catenated cell divisions, the amplification factor being about 1:16 for the granulocytic and erythrocytic cells. It is of great importance that these cells undergo a continuous process of maturation, the erythroblasts synthesizing more and more hemoglobin and the myelocytes maturing into granulocytes, characterized by a changing enzymatic pattern.

The most important cell pool in the hematopoietic cell-renewal system is the stem-cell pool, characterized by a capacity to release cells for differentiation, proliferation and maturation at a rate proportional to the loss of cells from the various pools of the system, particularly the functional pool, without exhausting itself. The hematopoietic stem-cell seems to have an indefinite capacity for replication, and there is no good evidence of aging in this system from intrinsic mechanisms (Lajtha and Schofield, 1971; Fliedner and Heit, 1975).

Of great importance for the understanding of cellular homeostasis in hema-topoietic cell-renewal systems is the functional structure of the stem-cell pool (Fliedner, 1975; Cronkite, 1975). This review is based on the concept of Stohl-man (1975) (Fig. 5). Myelopoiesis shares a common precursor cell with the erythroid and megakaryocytic elements which is known as the 'pluripotent hemopoietic stem cell' or colony-forming unit (CFU) (Till and McCulloch, 1961). Between the pluripotent stem cell and cells which can be identified under the light microscope as myeloid lies a compartment committed to myelopoiesis. Similar compartments are ready to respond with specific differentiation for erythropoiesis and megakaryocytopoiesis. Both monocytes and granulocytes are derived from a common precursor – the 'committed' myeloid stem cell. Fur-thermore, the myeloblast and promyelocyte may differentiate along one of 3 lines: neutrophil, basophil or eosinophil. As yet little is known as to at which stage (stem cell, myeloblast or promyelocyte) the transformation occurs, or about the factors controlling the development of specific cells.

The pluripotent stem-cell pool has been assayed in mice by the 'CFU assay' method developed by Till and McCulloch (1961). No comparable human test is yet available, but granulocytes, erythrocytes and megakaryocytes have been grown in diffusion chambers (Breivik et al., 1971; Bøyum et al., 1972; Cronkite et al., 1974).

The committed myeloid stem cell (CFUc) can be evaluated both in man and mice in the 'agar colony system' developed by Bradley and Metcalf (1966) and Pluznik and Sachs (1965). There is evidence that the myeloid progenitor cell

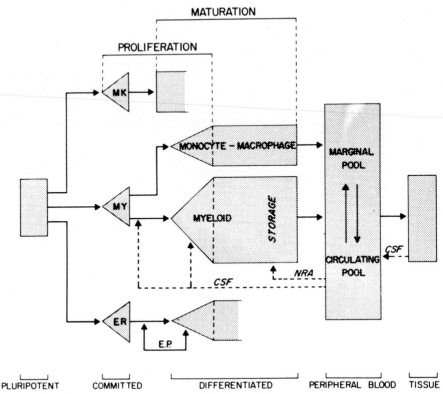

Fig. 5. Schematic representation of the hematopoietic stem-cell pool. MK = Megakaryopoietic stem cell; MY = Myelopoietic stem cell; ER = Erythropoietic stem cell; E.P. = Erythropoietin; CSF = Colony-stimulating factor; NRA = Neutrophil-releasing activity. From Stohlman Jr (1975); courtesy of the publishers.

grows and differentiates only when stimulated by a humoral factor, a colony-stimulating factor (CSF), probably produced by monocytes (Chervenik and LoBuglio, 1972), whereas granulocytes may be the source of a specific inhibitory factor (Shadduck, 1971; Heit et al., 1974).

Studies by Heit et al. (1975) show that there is no sharp boundary between the erythropoietic stem cells, as might be deduced from the concept of Stohlman (Fig. 5). In germ-free mice, these authors found evidence that spontaneous bone-marrow regeneration after whole-body irradiation occurred mainly in erythropoiesis and megakaryocytopoiesis and was greatly delayed in granulocytopoiesis. However, the administration of endotoxin rapidly produced granulocytopoiesis, though at the expense of erythropoiesis. On the other hand when irradiated germ-free mice are hypertransfused (to block erythropoietic differentiation), granulocytes rapidly appear.

Thus, although the 3 bone marrow-based cell lines are – in part – maintained and regulated independently, there is increasing evidence that this is only a partial autonomy. It now seems (see also review by Cronkite, 1975) that the stem-cell pool is a cell population with specified subpopulations responding to stimulating factors. In hypoxia caused by bleeding or high altitude, erythropoietin is produced which stimulates stem cells to produce red-cell precursors. The pluripotent stem cell is thought to be cytokinetically at rest under normal steady-state conditions and indistinguishable by light microscopy from a bone-marrow lymphocyte (Fliedner, 1975), but committed stem cells are largely 'in cycle', ready to respond to humoral stimulating factors such as erythropoietin (McCulloch and Till, 1970).

Thus, the hematopoietic cell-renewal systems have the most complex structure of the various cell systems so far reviewed. It must be remembered that all cell-renewal systems are bound to a supportive matrix: the connective tissue in the skin and mucous membranes and the bony capsule with the reticulum and endothelial cell matrix. In this context it may be recalled that in 1927 Askanazy alluded to the role of the bony capsule of the hematopoietic marrow and the fact that hematopoietic cells are parenchymal cells which eventually function some way from their home base and therefore require a greater degree of independence than other parenchymal cells. Both Fliedner et al. (1955) and Knospe et al. (1968) have emphasized the importance of the bone-marrow matrix, especially its sinusoid structure, in hematopoietic regeneration, and have referred to the environmental conditions which are essential for hematopoietic differentiation, as Trentin (1970) pointed out.

Regulatory mechanisms of cell systems

In the case of liver cell- and epithelial cell-renewal systems, some consideration has been given to the factors which seem to regulate them. In the liver, the loss of parenchymal cells (whether responsive or unresponsive G_0 cells), at least of 'non-dividing' cells, leads to a compensatory increase in cell production, which stops when the original mass has been restored. In the skin and mucous membranes, the loss of mature cells seems to be intimately connected with the stimulus of new production, which can also occur when the local concentration of an inhibiting factor decreases. In the mucous membranes, an increase in cell loss, not from the mature cells but rather from the dividing, and hence radiosensitive cells, after continuous exposure to low-level radiation, also results in a

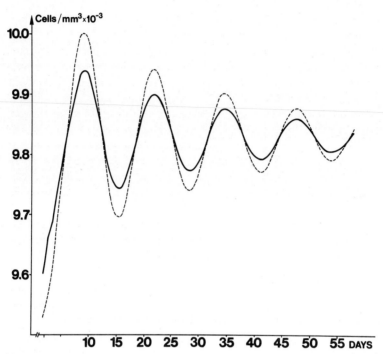

Fig. 6a. The theoretical response of granulocytes in the functional compartment of granulocytopoiesis following a single leukapheresis of 50% (solid line) and 75% (broken line) at t = 0 d. The granulocytes were previously assumed to be in a steady state at 9830 cells/mm^3.

compensatory increase in production, and after a certain time, a new steady state is established, although at a higher level of cell turnover.

Lamerton (1966) has clearly shown that this adaptive ability also holds true for hematopoiesis. If rats are irradiated with X-rays at a dose of 16 rads per day, the hemoglobin concentration remains normal for as long as 280 days. The platelets achieve a steady state after about 40 days and then remain constant. In the first 40 days there is great fluctuation, reflecting the efforts associated with the necessary compensatory actions. The mononuclear cells of the blood reach the lowest values after about 20 days and are normal thereafter, despite continued radiation. The polymorph count shows a transient reduction after about 20 days and then reaches normal or even above-normal values. When the ability of continuously irradiated cell systems to respond to stress situations was evaluated, a normal response pattern was found once the new steady-state equilibrium had been achieved. The incorporation of iron into red cells decreased when they

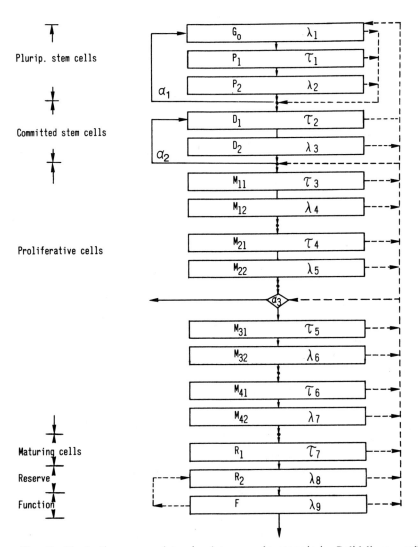

Fig. 6b. Block diagram used to simulate granulocytopoiesis. Solid lines = cell flow. Broken lines = information flow.

were injected into rats 3 weeks after the start of irradiation with 50 rads per day but returned to normal control values by 6 and 10 weeks. Removal of blood by phlebotomy 94 or 130 days after continuous irradiation with X-rays at a dosage of 50 rads per day did not impair the ability of the erythropoietic system to respond with regeneration at the same rate as in non-irradiated systems. Examination of the stem-cell pools provides evidence that the erythropoietic committed stem-cell pool seems to be intact after continuous irradiation, whereas the pluripotent stem-cell pool is drastically reduced. Thus, it may well be that the sensitivity of the entire hematopoietic system subjected to a continuing injury (such as radiation) is increased with respect to certain environmental factors. One may not be aware of such a burden for a long time. In such systems, further cytotoxic treatment may easily cause a sudden collapse of function.

Thus, it is possible that the most important factor in the regulation of cell-system activity – and thus the maintenance of cellular homeostasis – is the concentration or number of cells in the cell system. Normally, cells are removed from the functional pool at a rate determined by, among other factors, their utilization and aging. This triggers replacement and thus initiates a chain which – with decreasing impact – affects the respective precursor pools. Depending on various factors, such as the 'window-width' of cell concentration, e.g. for the granulocyte concentration in the blood, the lifespan of the cell, the storage pool characteristics, and the transit time for a cell to mature, one might expect cell-renewal systems to fluctuate as postulated by Morley et al. (1970). But even if no fluctuation can usually be found, one would expect to see damped fluctuation after a specific disturbance of the system.

The human granulocyte cell-renewal system has been used to simulate the effect of the sudden removal of a proportion of the circulating cells (Figs. 6a and b). The simulation language used was A S I M 2. Certain assumptions were made with respect to the cell kinetic parameters (Table 3). The blood-granulocyte concentration in this simulated granulocytic renewal system responded to the sudden withdrawal of 50% and 75% of the blood granulocytes (for example by leukapheresis) with a typical pattern of damped oscillations, the period of which was about 13 days, as could be predicted for a system with a transit time between the stem-cell level and the blood-granulocyte level of 6-7 days.

In a system such as that shown in Figure 6b, cell loss is seen as occurring at the level of the proliferating cells (α_3) or mature cells (F). Normally, the rate of cell loss may be small for the immature precursors compared with that of the mature ones from the blood. However, under continuous irradiation (as an extrinsic factor for cell damage) or in diseases such as leukemia, the rate of cell loss may already be so significant at the level of dividing-maturing cells that much fewer cells actually reach the blood. The system may then respond with increased production, but, because of a quantitative and/or qualitative defect in the cells at the stem-cell level, this is insufficient to compensate for the cell loss. Analysis of cytokinetic data from patients with acute leukemia by system simulation techniques shows that such an interpretation is possible (Fliedner et al., 1975).

TABLE 3

*Cell-cycle parameters used to simulate granulocytopoiesis
(about half what is actually found in man)*

Compartment	Number of cells	Transit time (hr)
G_0	800	$10,000 = 1/\lambda_1$
P_1	1.2	$15 = \tau_1$
P_2	0.4	$5 = 1/\lambda_2$
D_1	1,227.6	$15 = \tau_2$
D_2	409.2	$5 = 1/\lambda_3$
M_{11}	1,228.8	$15 = \tau_3$
M_{12}	409.6	$5 = 1/\lambda_4$
M_{21}	2,457.6	$15 = \tau_4$
M_{22}	819.2	$5 = 1/\lambda_5$
M_{31}	3,686.4	$15 = \tau_5$
M_{32}	1,228.8	$5 = 1/\lambda_6$
M_{41}	7,372.8	$15 = \tau_6$
M_{42}	2,457.6	$5 = 1/\lambda_7$
R_1	49,152	$50 = \tau_7$
R_2	49,152	$50 = 1/\lambda_8$
F	9.830.4	$10 = 1/\lambda_9$

In the controlled system α_1 is a function of cell number in the pluri-potent stem-cell pool, λ_1 and α_2 in the whole system, α_3 in R_2 and λ_8 in F. $\alpha_1 = 0.5$; $\alpha_2 = 0.499511241 = c.$ 10 divisions; $\alpha_3 = 0.75$.

Computer simulation of the blood-granulocyte labeling pattern after injection of tritiated thymidine into patients with acute leukemia demonstrates a rela-tionship between the granulocyte concentration in the blood and the inefficiency of cell production in the marrow. The findings are compatible with the assump-tion that in leukemia many cells that differentiate into promyelocytes rarely, if ever, divide, though they may mature while most of the cells die in the marrow. In leukemia, although the blood-granulocyte concentration is low, the system cannot respond with appropriate production.

Cellular homeostasis in cell-renewal systems

The purpose of this review has been to emphasize the role of cellular homeostasis in the maintenance of an equilibrium between cell removal and cell production. The various cell systems of the body differ widely in function, but they share some common structural characteristics and regulatory mechanisms. The most complex systems are those of hematopoiesis, with many different cell pools. The skin and mucous membranes represent much simpler systems, in which stem cells and proliferating cells are indistinguishable and feed directly into a functional pool. Last but not least, the liver is a system consisting only of a stem-cell pool, normally at rest but ready to respond at any time.

All these systems seem to be primarily regulated by cell loss, either from the functional pool alone or in combination with the dividing cell pool. If the stem-cell pool is intact, the system is ready to respond to small increases in cell loss with adequate compensatory mechanisms. If the stem-cell pool is not intact, e.g. after the action of cytotoxic agents or qualitative changes through malignant transformation, the maintenance of a homeostatic equilibrium depends on the capacity of the committed stem-cell pool.

The major regulatory mechanism of cell systems seems to be the presence of a sufficient concentration of an inhibitory factor, but there are long-range stimulatory factors acting directly at the stem-cell level, such as erythropoietin. The fine adjustment may be done by short-range factors, while the overall needs of the system are met through long-range factor activity.

Cell system physiology has made some advances in the last few years in trying to resolve some of the enigmas of cellular homeostasis, which is essential to the adaptation of the body to internal or external environmental changes. After studying cellular homeostasis one can only wonder at the miraculous mechanisms which enable the organism to make exact replicas of so many cells every day. In one lifetime, cellular homeostasis produces an almost incomprehensible number of cells without making any 'mistakes'. It is indeed surprising that more cells do not turn malignant or cease to function in normal man, though it may well be that such abnormal cells are produced but are dealt with by the organism's defense mechanisms.

References

Askanazy, M. (1927): In: *Handbuch der speziellen pathologischen Anatomie und Histologie, I, 2,* 775. Editors: F. Henkel and O. Lubarsch. Springer Verlag, Berlin.

Bond, V. P., Fliedner, T. M. and Archambeau, J. O. (1965): *Mammalian Radiation Lethality, a Disturbance of Cellular Kinetics.* Academic Press, New York-London.

Boylan, J. W. (Ed.) (1971): *Founders of Experimental Physiology.* J. F. Lehmanns Verlag, Munich.

Bøyum, A., Carsten, A. L., Laerum, O. D. and Cronkite, E. P. (1972): *Blood, 40,* 174.

Bradley, T. R. and Metcalf, D. (1966): *Aust. J. exp. Biol. med. Sci., 44,* 287.
Breivik, H., Benestad, H. B. and Bøyum, A. (1971): *J. Cell Physiol., 1,* 65.
Chervenik, P. A. and LoBuglio, A. F. (1972): *Science, 178,* 164.
Croft, D. N. and Cotton, P. B. (1973): *Digestion, 8,* 144.
Croft, D. N., Lins, C. C. and Taylor, J. F. N. (1968*a*): *Brit. J. Derm., 80,* 153.
Croft, D. N., Loehry, C. A. and Creamer, B. (1968*b*): *Lancet, 1,* 68.
Croft, D. N., Pollock, D. J. and Coghill, N. F. (1966): *Gut, 7,* 333.
Cronkite, E. P. (1975): In: *Pathobiology Annual,* p. 35. Editor: H. L. Joachim. Appleton-Century-Crofts, New York.
Cronkite, E. P., Boecker, W., Carsten, A. L., Chikkappa, G., Joel, D., Laissue, J. and Öhl, S. (1974): In: *Hemopoiesis in Culture,* p. 205. Editor: W. A. Robinson. U.S. Department of Health, Education and Welfare, No. NIH 74.
Fliedner, T. M. (1975): In: *Lymphozyt und klinische Immunologie.* Editors: H. Theml and H. Begemann. Springer-Verlag, Berlin – Heidelberg – New York.
Fliedner, T. M. and Heit, H. (1975): *Verh. dtsch. Ges. Path.*
Fliedner, T. M., Hoelzer, D. and Steinbach, K. H. (1975): *Brit. J. Haemat.,* submitted for publication.
Fliedner, T. M., Stodtmeister, R. and Sandkühler, S. (1955): *Z. zellforsch., 43,* 195.
Grundmann, E. (1969): In: *Handbuch der allgemeinen Pathologie VI/ II (Entwicklung, Wachstum).* Springer-Verlag, Berlin – Heidelberg – New York.
Heit, W., Heit, H., Kern, P. and Kubanek, B. (1975): *Radiat. Res.,* in press.
Heit, W., Kern, P., Heimpel, H. and Kubanek, B. (1974): *Blood, 44,* 511.
Hoelzer, D., Kurrle, E., Dietrich, M., Meyer-Hamme, K. D. and Fliedner, T. M. (1974): *Scand. J. Haemat., 12,* 311.
Hondius Boldingh, W. and Laurence, E. B. (1968): *Europ. J. Biochem., 5,* 191.
Iversen, O. H. (1969): In: *Homeostatic Regulators.* Editors: G. E. Wolstenholme and J. Knight. J. and A. Churchill Ltd., London.
Knospe, W. H., Blom, J. and Crosby, W. H. (1968): *Blood, 31,* 400.
Lajtha, L. G. and Schofield, R. (1971): *Geront. Res., 131,* 146.
Lamerton, L. F. (1966): *Radiat. Res., 27,* 119.
Lesher, S., Fry, R. J. M. and Sacher, G. A. (1961): *Exp. Cell Res., 25,* 398.
Lesher, S., Lamerton, L. F., Sacher, G. A., Fry, R. J. M., Gordon Steel, G. G. and Roylance, P. J. (1966): *Radiat. Res., 29,* 57.
Matsuzawa, T. and Wilson, R. (1965): *Radiat. Res., 25,* 15.
Maurer, H. R. (1973): *Z. Pharm. in neuer Zeit, 2,* 181.
McCulloch, E. A. and Till, J. E. (1970): In: *Hemopoietic Cellular Proliferation.* Editor: F. Stohlman. Grune and Stratton Inc., New York – London.
Morley, A., King-Smith, E. A. and Stohlman, F. (1970): In: *Hemopoietic Cellular Proliferation.* Editor: F. Stohlman. Grune and Stratton Inc., New York – London.
National Cancer Institute (1969): *Human Tumor Cell Kinetics.* Monograph 30, US Department of Health, Education and Welfare.
Nowicki, L., Martin, H. and Schubert, J. (Ed.) (1973): *Hämolyse – hämolytische Erkrankungen.* (Sonderbände zu *Blut, Band 11).* J. F. Lehmanns Verlag, Munich.
Oehlert, W. (1969): In: *Handbuch der allgemeinen Pathologie VI/ II.* Springer-Verlag, Berlin – Heidelberg – New York.
Pluznik, D. H. and Sachs, L. (1965): *J. cell. comp. Physiol., 66,* 319.
Rankin, R., Wilson, R. and Bealmear, P. M. (1971): *Proc. Soc. exp. Biol. (N. Y.), 138,* 270.

Rohrbach, R. (1975): In: *Veröffentlichungen aus der Pathologie, Heft 99*. Fischer Verlag, Stuttgart.

Saetren, H. (1956): *Exp. Cell Res., 11*, 229.

Shadduck, R. K. (1971): *Blood, 38*, 820.

Stack-Dunne, M. P. (1973): *Nat. Cancer Inst. Monogr., 38*, 185.

Stöcker, E., Schultze, B., Heine, W.-D. and Liebscher, H. (1972): *Z. Zellforsch., 125*, 306.

Stohlman Jr, F. (1975): In: *Prognostic Factors in Human Acute Leukemia*. Editors: T. M. Fliedner and S. Perry. Advances in the Biosciences 14, Pergamon Press, Oxford.

Till, J. E. and McCulloch, C. A. (1961): *Radiat. Res., 14*, 213.

Trentin, J. J. (1970): In: *Regulation of Hematopoiesis*. Editor: A. S. Gordon. Appleton-Century-Crofts, New York.

Trier, J. S. and Browning, T. H. (1970): *New Engl. J. Med., 283*, 1245.

Verly, W. G., Deschamps, J., Pushpathadam, J. and Desrosiers, M. (1971): *Canad. J. Biochem., 49*, 1376.

Weiss, P. and Kavanau, J. L. (1957): *J. gen. Physiol., 41*, 1.

2: Inborn disease

Defective genes

C. R. Scriver

*The deBelle Laboratory for Biochemical Genetics, Medical Research
Council Group in Medical Genetics, Departments of Pediatrics and Biology,
Faculties of Medicine and Science, McGill University, Montreal, Canada*

An exponential increase in the publication rate of papers dealing with new
observations in human genetics has characterized the medical sciences in recent
years (Childs, 1967). However, this evidence of a discipline being alive and well is
not necessarily reflected in recognition gained either by the establishment of new
departments of genetics within universities, or in the teaching of genetics to
medical students (Childs, 1974). Accordingly, the emphasis given to human and
medical genetics at the Ninth World Congress of the World Association of
Societies of Pathology is welcome.

With its emphasis on aberration, the title of this paper might divert one from
recognizing an important feature of 'normal' human genes, namely their great
diversity and variability. One might readily ask whether this characteristic,
sustained as it is by mutation, is an indication of defectiveness. We must begin,
then, by examining the nature of interindividual genetic variation, which is a
major biological attribute of mankind, and is responsible not only for our
heritage, but also for all that is uniquely human.

Let me begin with Thomas Hardy, the novelist and poet who championed

Charles Darwin within months of the publication of *The Origin of Species*, and who believed in 'evolutionary meliorism' or what we would now call homological evolution, meaning the process whereby man improves his relationship with the environment and thus influences his own evolution. Shortly after Mendel's original description of genes had been translated into English by Bateson (1902), Hardy responded with a haunting poem entitled *Heredity:*

> I am the family face;
> Flesh perishes, I live on
> Projecting trait and trace
> Through time to times anon,
> And leaping from place to place
> Over oblivion.

Hardy speaks of those features which inform us about faces in the crowd.

In her own way, the late Diane Arbus, who was an unsettling photographer of human aberrations, also pulled some messages out of the crowd. The photograph of identical twins which appeared on the cover of her posthumous portfolio said, in the language of Arbus, that twins are not the usual way we humans go about reproducing ourselves. Arbus believed that to be identical to someone else is a form of private trauma.

The striking similarity in bodily features evident in monozygotic twins is apparent even in the multifactorial metabolic events which regulate, for example, their plasma amino acid levels (Scriver and Rosenberg, 1973). Dizygotic twins have more discordant plasma amino acid levels and physical features; nonsibs are yet more different from each other. From twins we learn that the genetic control of morphogenetic and metabolic events, which make us individuals, is pervasive. The fact that the frequency of monozygotic twins in the human species is only 3.5-4 per 1000 live births means that nearly all human beings have dissimilar genomes and that interindividual genetic heterogeneity will be more the rule than the exception. In this sense we are very different from prime specimens of cattle or corn where constant and predictable genetic content of the organism is a virtue and an asset for the breeder or planter.

Sir Archibald Garrod collected, not poetic or photographic impressions, but chemical impressions of odd people. He too honored the odd man out, the 'sport' among us, and from his probings came the great theme of human chemical individuality (Garrod, 1902). The concluding paragraph of Garrod's extraordinary paper on alcaptonuria contains these ideas, far in advance of their time:

> 'If it be indeed the case that in alkaptonuria ... we are dealing with (an) individuality of metabolism ..., the thought naturally presents itself that (it is)

a merely extreme example of variation of chemical behaviour ... elsewhere present in minor degrees, and that ... just as no two individuals of a species are absolutely identical in bodily structure, neither are their chemical processes carried out on exactly the same lines. ... Again, in their behaviour to different drugs and infecting organisms the members of the various genera and species manifest peculiarities which presumably have a chemical basis ...'

Location, quantity and origin of genetic diversity in man

The assignment of specific genes to physical locations (loci) on human chromosomes has until recently been a very slow and difficult task. However, the advent of methods for cell hybridization and complementation analysis (Ruddle, 1972) has made more feasible the systematic assignment of specific genes to linked clusters of gene loci (syntenic groups) and to actual human chromosomes or parts of chromosomes. Nonetheless, even by these methods, assignment with confirmation is proceeding at the slow rate of about only one gene locus per month; accordingly, it will be many years before the full human genome is mapped in any way comparable to the achievement in mouse genetics. Moreover, the physical mapping of gene loci in man will not reveal the allelic variation (different forms of a gene) that may exist at these loci between individuals.

The systematic use of electrophoresis as a means of analyzing compositional differences in proteins (gene products) has enabled various investigators to make estimates of the extent of genetic diversity between individuals at several specific gene loci. All cellular and extracellular functions, from those determined by structural proteins (the collagens and keratins, for example) to those served by catalysts of chemical conversion and transport reactions (enzymes and transport proteins), are performed by one or another specific protein. Our proteins are the true reflection of the genetic diversity between individuals and they determine our chemical individuality, as it was originally perceived by Garrod.

The amount of interindividual variation in the human genome is impressive. Harris and colleagues, who pioneered studies of 'normal' variation, examined a profile of several enzymes in blood cells and plasma (Harris and Hopkinson, 1972). They observed that at least 1% of persons have an inherited variant of the enzymes specified by 28% of the 71 structural gene loci they examined; the average heterozygosity per locus was 0.067. Because noteworthy frequencies of variability were in fact found for all of the enzymes that they studied by electrophoresis, it seems likely that these frequencies are underestimates of the true incidence and extent of genetic variation at human gene loci. From these and many following studies, it was recognized that variability at a given locus and expressed in more than 1% of the population is the normal situation. Genes responsible for this degree of variation in their protein products are said to be 'polymorphic' (Harris and Hopkinson, 1972; Cannings and Cavalli-Sforza, 1973).

Mutation is the ultimate source of the variation in DNA composition between individuals. The continuing occurrence of new mutations, and the accumulation of past mutations, has yielded the variable genome which characterizes modern man. Mutation usually involves the substitution of one nucleotide for another in a DNA molecule, with the complementary change appearing in the paired nucleotide during synthesis of the homologous DNA strand. Nucleotide substitutions, or deletions and insertions with the subsequent frame shifts in translation of the DNA sequence, constitute the simplest form of mutation. More complex and massive changes can also occur with translocation, duplication, or inversion of larger sequences of DNA, or even of entire chromosome segments. The various haptoglobin types (Sutton, 1970), for example, clearly illustrate the important role of gene duplication in the evolution of human proteins.

The rate of mutation is a matter of constant concern and its measurement is a complicated discipline (Edwards, 1974). Most workers would agree, however, that the general frequency of mutation in man is on the average lower than 10^{-5} per gene locus per generation. Consequently, only 10 to 100 nucleotide pair differences per individual arise from 'new' mutation affecting parental gametes. Clearly, this mutation rate is insufficient to explain the much greater heterozygosity per gene locus which characterizes man (Harris and Hopkinson, 1972). As it happens, the load of mutations we now carry is related to their effects.

Three effects of mutation can be envisaged (Cannings and Cavalli-Sforza, 1973) (Fig. 1). The mutant gene may be harmful (a 'defective' gene so as to reduce genetic fitness); it may have no apparent effect in the customary environment (a 'neutral' mutation with indeterminant effect on fitness); or it may be beneficial, enhancing fitness. Natural selection largely influences the frequency of genes with the first and the last characteristic; random genetic drift largely determines the frequency of the neutral mutation. The relative frequency of a neutral mutation will increase entirely by random chance (genetic drift) in the second generation in populations where it is customary to have multiple progeny (Fig. 1). Repetition of the increase by chance through successive generations can bring the frequency of a mutant gene to a very high level, even to the point where all individuals will carry it. For example, in the case of L-gulonic acid dehydrogenase deficiency, man is apparently isogenic for this defect in L-ascorbic acid synthesis (Burns, 1959). In an environment providing adequate dietary vitamin C, this mutation is neutral and the isogenic status will be the result of random

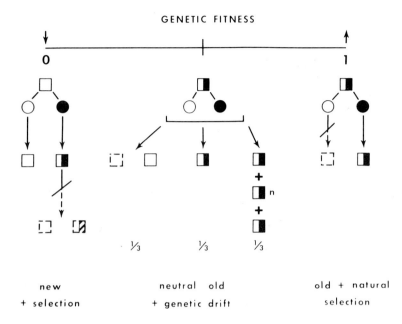

GENETIC FITNESS

0   1

1/3   1/3   1/3

new   neutral   old   old + natural

+ selection   + genetic drift   selection

Fig. 1. Interaction between mutation and environment (natural selection *vs.* genetic drift) and effect on frequency of genes. Mutation can be disadaptive causing reduced genetic fitness (0 end of scale) or beneficial (1 end of scale). A 'new' disadaptive mutation (left side) in the gamete (circles) causes reduced fitness in proband (squares), and because of natural selection is passed on with low (or zero) frequency. An 'old' advantageous mutation (right side) benefits proband; such individuals are selected to pass on the gene while those without this mutational advantage may not actually survive to pass on the 'normal' gene. Most 'old' mutations are neutral and polymorphic. Random genetic drift (excluding 'founder' effect) largely determines the frequency of neutral mutations. The proband (carrier of the gene) may have no children or not pass on the mutation to offspring, or the gene is passed on, but only to one child, or it is passed on to more than one child. In growing populations with multiple offspring per parent, the relative frequency of neutral mutations will increase by random chance.

genetic drift without the invocation of any selective advantage (or disadvantage) for it.

Mutations which are harmful, or disadvantageous, are the proper domain of medical genetics, but what of advantageous mutation? Physicians and pathologists, who inevitably experience a bias in their predominant exposure to harmful mutation, tend to consider mutation in general to be harmful. The classical example of a mutant gene which has actually enhanced genetic fitness under certain conditions is that causing sickle or S hemoglobin ($\beta_6$glu → val). Hemoglobin S confers some resistance to infection of the erythrocyte with *Plasmodium falciparum*. Thus, in a malarial environment the heterozygous carrier of the sickle cell mutation is better protected from falciparum malaria and does not experience the disadvantage of sickle cell disease. The selective advantage for carriers of the sickle hemoglobin gene in a malarial region and the autosomal recessive inheritance pattern of this gene combine to yield an approximate relative frequency of 18:1 for heterozygotes relative to mutant homozygotes with the disease among populations in malarial regions where the typical S gene frequency is about 10%. Under such conditions of gene-environment interaction, approximately one-fifth of persons have become carriers of the seemingly harmful S mutation.

In summary, it is apparent that the human genome comprises many mutations: some are harmful; a few are clearly beneficial under certain environmental (or selective) conditions; while most are apparently neutral, their effect undeclared or unknown in the customary human situation. The disadvantageous expression of mutation may be clearly apparent as monogenic disease (or disadaptation); more often it is expressed under more complex (multifactorial) conditions.

Cellular expression of mutation

Garrod (1902) studied aberrant metabolic processes as a reflection of single-gene variation. The metabolic aberration is, however, one step removed, or more, from the action of the mutant gene product. If the normal enzyme exerts its action outside the cell, the mutant event will also be extracellular, as for example the blood clotting abnormality with factor VIII deficiency in classical hemophilia. More often, the event is intracellular and there are many mechanisms by which mutant gene products can express themselves in the cell (Fig. 2).

The enzyme may normally act in the cytoplasm; the cytosol enzyme is the traditional domain of the inborn error of metabolism. However, as shown by studies of β-glucuronidase activity in mice (Paigen, 1961), mutation may affect a binding site at which the enzyme acts in the cell.

Garrod proposed that cystinuria was an inborn error of cystine metabolism. Some 50 years later, Dent and Harris (1951) showed that this trait and others resembling it were inborn errors of membrane transport. Mutations which affect the membrane transport proteins and lead to disturbances in cellular uptake and

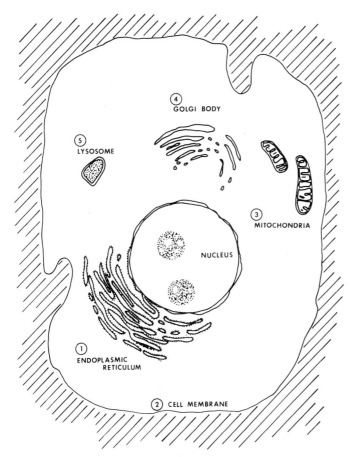

GOLGI BODY

LYSOSOME

MITOCHONDRIA

NUCLEUS

ENDOPLASMIC
RETICULUM

CELL MEMBRANE

Fig. 2. Possible intracellular sites for expression of mutant catalytic functions. They include: (1) cytoplasmic enzymes (and binding sites); (2) membrane transport processes (and surface recognition sites, etc); (3) mitochondrial functions; (4) biosynthetic glycosylation activities; (5) degradative lysosomal activities. Mutant genes can also be expressed in structural (non-catalytic) proteins (intracellular and extracellular), and through extracellular catalytic functions (e.g. transport of substances in blood, blood clotting, etc.)

regulation of cellular fuels and constituents result in an important class of disorders in their own right (Scriver and Hechtman, 1970).

Compartmentation of cellular events is an important aspect of the packaging of biological functions. Delineation of intra-mitochondrial mutant enzymes was merely a matter of time; investigation of the hereditary diseases of the urea cycle

(Scriver and Rosenberg, 1973; Shih and Efron, 1972) reveals that those affecting the synthesis of citrulline are limited to the mitochondrion, while others, concerned with disposal of citrulline and formation of urea from arginine, exist in the cytoplasm. Many enzymes exist as isozymes, one form being active in the cytoplasm, another in mitochondria. Cytosol tyrosine aminotransferase deficiency is an example of an inborn error of metabolism in which the cytoplasmic tyrosine transamination activity is deficient, while the mitochondrial isozyme is intact (Fellman et al., 1969).

The Golgi apparatus is largely responsible for glycosylation of proteins. The biochemical genetics of the blood groups (Watkins, 1967) may, in part, be the result of gene expression through activity of the Golgi body. A recently described disease affecting GM_3 ganglioside biosynthesis (Fishman et al., 1975) is likely to be an inborn error of Golgi body glycosylation activity.

Many cellular products end their biological life in the lysosome; defective intra-lysosomal enzyme activity will lead to storage of precursor debris in the lysosomes, which will then hypertrophy. The various storage diseases involving gangliosides, mucopolysaccharide material and glycogen, for example, reflect the mutant expression of genes controlling various acid hydrolases in lysosomes (Neufeld, 1974).

The pathologist can often recognize the specific cellular effects of the various classes of mutant genes by the appropriate fixation, staining and examination of biopsy or necropsy material. For example, it was the cytoplasmic rather than the lysosomal deposition of GM_3 ganglioside which lead to the delineation of the first disease of ganglioside biosynthesis (Fishman et al., 1975) as distinct from a disorder of GM_3 ganglioside catabolism.

The nature of genetic disease

The fourth edition (1975) of McKusick's catalogue of inheritance in man lists 2336 Mendelian traits, many of which are associated with disease states in our customary human environment. However, to view genetic disease in man only as monogenic in origin would be too narrow a perspective. Much genetic disease is multigenic and multifactorial (with both environmental and genetic factors interacting under defined conditions). Indeed, there is a spectrum of disease (Fig. 3) with causes extending from the clearly genetic to the clearly environmental. The aggregate number of the 'rare' genetic diseases is large even if their individual frequency is low. On the other hand, many of the 'common' diseases of man are multifactorial in their pathogenesis, and multigenic in their inherited component.

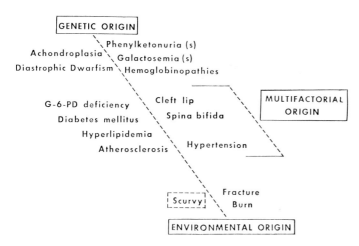

Fig. 3. A spectrum of disease ranging from those of primarily monogenic origin to those of primarily environmental origin. (Note that the isogenic mutation in man affecting ascorbic acid synthesis is apparent only in an environment deficient in ascorbic acid.) Many ecogenetic traits with particular gene-environment relationships and many common diseases of multigenic and multifactorial origin occupy the middle of the spectrum.

The expression of monogenic diseases can take form as either inborn errors of 'enzyme proteins' (Harris, 1968) producing disorders of metabolism, such as galactosemia, or as inborn errors of 'structural proteins' producing disorders of morphogenesis (Holllmes, 1974) such as achondroplasia. However, within any given form of expression, the occurrence of genetic heterogeneity (Childs and Der Kaloustian, 1968) must again be considered. Mutant genes may occur in several different forms (alleles). For example, Sickle hemoglobin is but one of the variant proteins produced by mutation at the β-chain locus. Different alleles at this gene locus produce a variety of mutant β-chains and consequently a variety of β-chain hemoglobinopathies (Perutz and Lehmann, 1968); the same gene is affected in each, but the alleles and their effect are different one from another. Phenylketonuria is but one of several forms of hereditary hyper-phenylalaninemia in man (Scriver and Rosenberg, 1973), each representing a different mutation at one or more gene locus controlling phenylalanine hydroxylation activity. Galactosemia (Segal, 1972; Tedesco et al., 1975) is the result of three different types of mutation at three separate gene loci controlling galactokinase, galactose-1-phosphate uridylyl transferase and UDPgalactose-4-epimerase activity respectively; it is also the result of several mutant alleles at one of these loci as revealed by the several forms of transferase deficiency which have been described as 'classical', Duarte and Negro variants for example. The manifestations of heterogeneity are no less in the inborn errors of morphogenesis. For example, achondroplasia is dominantly inherited, and diastrophic dwarfism, which resembles it at first glance, is an altogether different mutation inherited as an autosomal recessive at a different locus. Accordingly, the pathologist must be alert to genetic heterogeneity in the mutant state since it will be relevant to the diagnosis, prognosis, treatment and counselling of the proband and family.

More subtle are the mutations which express themselves only under certain conditions of environment. Such individuals may be considered 'normal' until their genetic status is declared upon exposure to a particular drug, food, inhalant or 'physical' agent (Table 1). These 'ecogenetic' phenomena (Omenn and Motulsky, 1975) may come to be an increasingly important component of late-onset disease as we learn to appreciate better how our own particular interaction with the environment is determined by our 'silent' and often polymorphic genes. The pharmacogenetic variants are the best known, present-day examples of these health problems.

The group of diseases in the middle of the spectrum (Fig. 3) require special consideration (see Carter, *This Volume*). This is the domain of the common 'degenerative' diseases of later onset in life. Important environmental components exist in each, but genetic predispositions are present also; hence their multifactorial classification. Moreover, with respect to pathological states such as atherosclerosis and the antecedent hyperlipidemias, there may be several genes involved in the (multigenic) origin of the condition in a population.

The hyperlipidemias are a useful model to illustrate the concepts underlying multigenic origins of disease. If we consider, for example, the distribution of the blood cholesterol concentration among individuals in a population, we would expect discontinuous variation with a bimodal distribution of values (Fig. 4) if hypercholesterolemia were the result of only a single mutation. However, a unimodal distribution (quasicontinuous variation) could exist if several mutant genes caused hypercholesterolemia and several additional genes were responsible for normal cholesterol metabolism. Goldstein et al. (1973a, b) adopted the hypothesis that hyperlipidemia was an important predisposing factor in early-onset coronary (ischemic) heart disease. They believe that monogenic forms of hyperlipidemia are expressed in 54% of the hyperlipidemic survivors of myocardial infarction under 60 years of age. By means of genetic studies, they believe they can discern three different mutant genes involved in this cohort of patients; that each is inherited as an autosomal dominant; and that between 0.6 and 1.0% of the general population carried these genes. In other words, a small fraction of the general population at birth becomes a major fraction of those with hyper-

TABLE 1

*Some host-environment (ecogenetic) relationships**

Environmental agent	Clinical response	Mutant host function
Drugs		
Oxidant drugs	Hemolysis	Glucose-6-phosphate dehydrogenase
Acetylated drugs	Neuropathy	N-acetyltransferase
Methemoglobin-forming drugs	Cyanosis	Methemoglobin reductase
Suxamethonium	Paralysis (transient)	Pseudocholinesterase (at least 33 mutant alleles)
Foods		
Lactose	Diarrhea	Intestinal lactose
Gluten (α-Gliaden)	Celiac disease	Unknown (associated with histocompatibility genotype)
Cholesterol	Coronary heart disease	Low-density lipoprotein membrane receptor (and other factors)
Fava beans	Hemolysis	Glucose-6-phosphate dehydrogenase
Goitrogens	Goitre	Phenylthiocarbamide taste perception
Chocolate and cheese	Migraine	Monoamine oxidase
Caffeine	Insomnia	CNS receptor
Inhalants		
Cigarette smoke	Lung cancer	Arylhydrocarbon hydroxylase
	Emphysema	? α_1-antitrypsin
Nicotine	Bladder cancer	Cotinine: nicotine-l'N-oxide ratio
Physical		
UV radiation	Xeroderma pigmentosum	DNA repair (several loci)
Color	Color blindness	Deutan, protan series
Infections		
Pl. falciparum	Malaria	Hemoglobin S (β-locus)
Virus	Diabetes spondylitis	HL-A histocompatibility type

* Adapted from Omenn and Motulsky (1975). Definition of ecogenetic: 'genetically determined differences among individuals in their susceptibility to the action of environmental agents' (Omenn and Motulsky, 1975).

Frequency

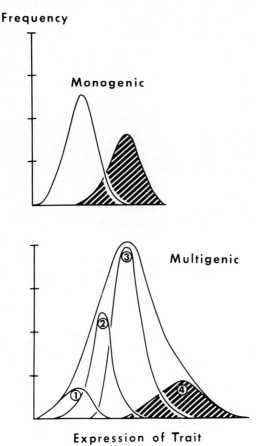

Expression of Trait

Fig. 4. Trait of monogenic origin exhibiting bimodal variation, and trait of multigenic origin exhibiting quasicontinuous variation.

lipidemic ischemic heart disease. Whereas it has yet to be proven that prospective treatment and change of lifestyle will reduce the risk of heart disease in those at specific risk, it is quite evident that delineation of the owners of the hyperlipidemia genes yields the appropriate candidates for research on the specific role of preventive treatment and that the major fraction of the population can avoid conscription into such studies. Furthermore, the genetic approach rationalizes the empiric evidence that the different types of hyperlipidemia need different forms of treatment (Levy et al., 1974).

The amount of disease due to defective gene expression

Estimates of disease caused by aberrant gene expression in the fetus, among live births, and in childhood are beginning to reveal the size of the burden. Major malformations, which appear during intrauterine morphogenesis, often as the result of post-fertilization chromosomal aberrations comprise the majority of first trimester spontaneous abortions (Poland and Lowry, 1974). Rejection of the deformed product of conception appears then to be an important mechanism for the disposal of genetic errors in the human species.

The recent findings of Trimble and Doughty (1974), derived from multiple-input ascertainment of handicapping disease in a defined population, update earlier and more general data assembled by a World Health Organization Expert Committee (1972) and reveal the extent of defective gene expression among live births. At least 180 individuals per 100,000 live births are born with diseases of single-gene cause. This frequency will vary between different geographic and demographic regions as the result of gene segregation and 'founder effects' (Cannings and Cavalli-Sforza, 1973; World Health Organization, 1972). Consequently, this figure might easily be doubled in some parts of the world. At least another 160 persons per 100,000 live births will have chromosomal anomalies, and again the frequency will vary, in particular according to the prevailing maternal age in the population. For example, the rate for trisomy-21 (Down's syndrome) will rise if the average maternal age at conception is advanced, and again the rate might be doubled in some regions. Congenital malformations of multifactorial origin will occur in another 3580 births according to the study of Trimble and Doughty (1974), while another 1580 persons are estimated, in their study, to be born with diseases with some genetic content. These estimates are considered to be conservative; nonetheless, they are sufficient to indicate that at least 1 in 20 humans is born with a major handicapping condition of partial or wholly genetic cause.

The 'fallout' of these births into the world's hospitals is also impressive. Several studies (Childs et al., 1972; Scriver et al., 1973; Day and Holmes, 1973) indicate that up to 30% of pediatric hospital admissions are of the above-mentioned types of illness. In my own hospital, for example (Scriver et al., 1973), single-gene diseases account for 6.9% of admissions; common multigenic problems are another 3.8%, while chromosomal disease is 0.4%. The aggregate comprises about 10% of admissions. Another 18.5% of admissions is composed of common and rare multifactorial congenital malformations, bringing the total admission rate due to defective gene expression to about 30%. The corresponding mortality data (Carter, 1956; Roberts et al., 1970) reveal that in excess of 40% of pediatric deaths in hospitals are the result of defective gene expression.

Modifying of the impact of defective genes

Two primary approaches will alleviate harmful expression of mutant genes in man: either the mutation may be avoided altogether by preventing the birth of the affected proband (negative eugenics); or the expression of the gene may be neutralized by modifying the host's environment (euthenic approach).

Numerous preventive modes exist in medical genetics (Scriver, 1972; Clow et al., 1973) to serve the individual and society. One of the important and newest options is genetic screening (National Academy of Sciences, 1975), the objectives of which are: to provide the opportunity for medical intervention through case finding and diagnosis; to provide the opportunity for reproductive counselling; and to permit enumeration (and delineation) by means of epidemiologic and research methods. The screening activity may be directed at a major subgroup of the population (e.g. all newborn infants), in which case it is mass screening, or at selected subgroups (e.g. an ethnic component, or a deme), when it is called selective screening. In the particular context of medical genetics, the screening may be directed at the proband, that is at a person with, or at risk for, a genetic disease, or it may seek out non-probands who are themselves at no risk but who carry genes which, if inherited by their offspring in a particular fashion, could cause disease in the latter. Screening for hyperphenylalaninemia in the newborn population is an example of proband-oriented, mass screening with case finding followed by diagnosis for purposes of medical intervention to prevent mental retardation caused by phenylketonuria. Screening for carriers of the Tay-Sachs gene is an example of selective screening among healthy non-probands for purposes of reproductive counselling to prevent the birth of affected homozygotes. Screening for the monogenic hyperlipidemias at the present time might be either selective or mass in scope; it is presumably proband oriented; and it is clearly epidemiologic in structure unless the objective is to pursue research on the prevention of ischemic heart disease by means of long-term clinical trials.

The timing of the modifying intervention is of great importance. For handicapping diseases without effective postnatal treatment the negative eugenic intervention must occur before the birth of the child to reduce the burden of such illness. The imposition on parents is severe when the constraints are upon conception itself. Where somatic cell genetics and other methods permit prenatal classification (diagnosis) of the fetal genotype in the mid-trimester, it is possible to offer the parents the option of pregnancy termination when the fetus is an affected proband, and continuation of the pregnancy when it is not affected. The benefits of prenatal diagnosis to couples with a fetus at risk are apparent.

Conditions which respond to postnatal treatment require a reliable structure of case finding, diagnosis and intervention so that probands are found before expression of the mutant allele takes its toll (National Academy of Sciences, 1975). The benefit to society and to individuals in this type of genetics program and the cost of such activities are the subject of ongoing evaluation (National Academy of Sciences, 1975).

Finally, the prevention of gene expression in later life, as for example in ecogenetic circumstances, is of increasing interest in those societies where reduction of total disease burden, and cost, is an important objective in the application of the health budget.

The euthenic approach to phenotype modification is largely confined to the hereditary metabolic disorders (monogenic and multigenic). Several environmental mechanisms (Fig. 5) can be used to offset the effects of mutant genes (Clow et al., 1973). They include: (1) substrate restriction by dietary means, or by the imposition of artificial blocks at alternate points in pathways, or by removal of toxic metabolites; (2) product replacement, if deficiency of the metabolite normally produced by the mutant reaction causes disease; (3) amplification of residual enzyme activity by vitamin (coenzyme) supplementation; and (4) enzyme replacement itself. In the last of these approaches, knowledge of the mutant enzyme with respect to the immunological status of cross-reacting material is essential (Scriver, 1974; Boyer et al., 1973). Infusion of normal enzyme into a

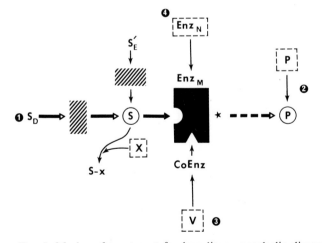

Fig. 5. Modes of treatment for hereditary metabolic disease including: (1) substrate restriction (if substrate accumulation is toxic); (2) product replacement (to offset a deficiency state); (3) enzyme enhancement by coenzyme supplementation (vitamin-responsive hereditary metabolic disease); and (4) enzyme replacement.

cross-reacting material-negative mutant subject will provoke grave immuno-
logic intolerance. Thus the immunopathology of mutant enzymes has come to
be of as much practical significance as a knowledge of diets and chemical agents
for the therapeutic management of hereditary metabolic disease.

Comment

Concern for genetic disease will become a global issue. Nations with high birth
rates now have, as it were, a mechanism to offset the effect of disease which
depletes the youthful population; reproductive compensation sustains a pool of
genes to pass on to the next generation. In such countries, now, the relative
importance of genetic disease is diminished. However, in the demographic transition from agrarian to post-industrial society characteristic of developing nations now and in the future, their birth rate will drop; the presence of genetic
disease in human affairs will then achieve a prominence that cannot be ignored.
Moreover, with fewer conceptions per parent, each will be more crucial to the
family and will demand all the benefits of new genetic knowledge. Thus our
concerns of today are very relevant to the immediate future of mankind in all
nations.

All progress comes at a price. Thomas Hardy, in a letter to a friend, said:

What we gain by science is, after all, sadness. The more we know of the laws
and nature of the universe, the more ghastly a business one perceives it all to
be.

Perhaps we can let ourselves believe that the appropriate application of the
new knowledge about our greatest human resource, namely our genetic diversity, will enhance our personal dignity where, otherwise, we might seem to face an
inhospitable society and a ghastly universe as ciphers.

Acknowledgements

I am grateful to F. Clarke Fraser who is constantly teaching me more about human
genetics and to Huguette Ishmael and Lynne Prevost for assistance in the preparation of
this manuscript.

References

Bateson, W. (1902): *Mendel's Principles of Heredity*. Cambridge University Press, London.

Boyer, S. H., Siggers, D. C. and Krueger, L. J. (1973): *Lancet, 2,* 654.

Burns, J. J. (1959): *Amer. J. Med., 26,* 740.

Cannings, C. and Cavalli-Sforza, L. (1973): *Advanc. hum. Genet., 4,* 105.

Carter, C. O. (1956): *Gt Ormond Str. J., 11,* 65.

Childs, B. (1967): *Amer. J. Dis. Child., 114,* 467.

Childs, B. (1974): *Amer. J. hum. Genet., 26,* 120.

Childs, B. and Der Kaloustian, M. (1968): *New Engl. J. Med., 279,* 1205 and 1267.

Childs, B., Miller, S. M. and Bearn, A. G. (1972): In: *Mutagenic Effects of Environmental Contamination*, p. 3. Editors: H. E. Sutton and M. I. Harris. Academic Press, New York.

Clow, C. L., Fraser, F. C., Laberge, C. and Scriver, C. R. (1973): *Progr. med. Genet. 9,* 159.

Day, N. and Holmes, L. B. (1973): *Amer. J. hum. Genet., 25,* 237.

Dent, C. E. and Harris, H. (1951): *Ann. Eugen. (Lond.), 16,* 60.

Edwards, J. H. (1974): *Progr. med. Genet., 10,* 1.

Fellman, J. H., Vanbellinghen, P. J., Jones, R. T. and Koler, R. D. (1969): *Biochemistry, 8,* 615.

Fishman, P. H., Max, S. R., Tallman, J. F., Brady, R. O., MacLaren, N. K. and Cornblath, M. (1975): *Science, 187,* 68.

Garrod, A. E. (1902): *Lancet, 2,* 1616.

Goldstein, J. L., Hazzard, W. R., Schrott, H. G., Bierman, E. L. and Motulsky, A. G. (1973a): *J. clin. Invest., 52,* 1533.

Goldstein, J. L., Schrott, H. G., Hazzard, W. R., Bierman, E. L. and Motulsky, A. G. (1973b): *J. clin. Invest., 52,* 1544.

Harris, H. (1968): *Brit. Med. J., 1,* 135.

Harris, H. and Hopkinson, D. A. (1972): *Ann. hum. Genet., 36,* 9.

Holmes, L. B. (1974): *New Engl. J. Med., 291,* 763.

Levy, R. I., Morganroth, J. and Rifkin, B. M. (1974): *New Engl. J. Med., 290,* 1295.

McKusick, V. A. (1975): *Mendelian Inheritance in Man, 4th ed.* Johns Hopkins Press, Baltimore.

National Academy of Sciences (1975): *Genetic Screening*. Washington, P.C.

Neufeld, E. F. (1974): *Progr. med. Genet., 10,* 81.

Omenn, G. S. and Motulsky, A. G. (1975): In: *Genetics and Public Health*. Editor: B. Cohen. Johns Hopkins University Press, Baltimore, in press.

Paigen, K. (1961): *Exp. Cell Res., 25,* 286.

Perutz, M. F. and Lehmann, H. (1968): *Nature (Lond.), 219,* 902.

Poland, J. B. and Lowry, R. B. (1974): *Amer. J. Obstet. Gynec., 118,* 322.

Roberts, D. F., Chavez, J. and Court, S. D. M. (1970): *Arch. Dis. Childh., 45,* 33.

Ruddle, F. H. (1972): *Advanc. hum. Genet., 3,* 173.

Scriver, C. R. (1972): In: *Proceedings, IV International Congress of Human Genetics, Paris, 1971*, p. 10. Editor: J. de Grouchy. ICS 250. Excerpta Medica, Amsterdam.

Scriver, C. R. (1974): In: *Proceedings, IV International Conference on Birth Defects*, p. 114. Editors: A. G. Motulsky and W. Lentz. ICS 310. Excerpta Medica, Amsterdam.

Scriver, C. R. and Hechtman, P. (1970): *Advanc. hum. Genet., 1,* 211.

Scriver, C. R., Neal, J. L., Saginur, R. and Clow, A. (1973): *Canad. med. Ass. J., 108,* 1111.

Scriver, C. R. and Rosenberg, L. E. (1973): *Amino Acid Metabolism and its Disorders.* W. B. Saunders, Philadelphia.

Segal, S. (1972): In: *The Metabolic Basis of Inherited Disease, 3rd ed.,* p. 174. Editors: J. B. Stanbury, J. B. Wyngaarden and D. S. Fredrickson. McGraw-Hill, New York.

Shih, V. E. and Efron, M. L. (1972): In: *The Metabolic Basis of Inherited Disease, 3rd ed.,* p. 374. Editors: J. B. Stanbury, J. B. Wyngaarden and D. S. Frederickson. McGraw-Hill, New York.

Sutton, H. E. (1970): *Progr. med. Genet., 7,* 163.

Tedesco, T. A., Wu, J. W., Boches, F. S. and Mellman, W. J. (1975): *New Engl. J. Med., 292,* 737.

Trimble, B. K. and Doughty, J. H. (1974): *Ann. hum. Genet., 38,* 199.

Watkins, W. M. (1967): In: *Proceedings, III International Congress of Human Genetics,* p. 171. Editors: J. F. Crow and J. V. Neel. Johns Hopkins Press, Baltimore.

World Health Organization (1972): *Wld Hlth Org. techn. Rep. Ser.,* 497.

Foetal damage

H. Tuchmann-Duplessis

Laboratoire d'Embryologie, Faculté de Médecine, Paris, France

The two main teratological discoveries in recent times were made in Australia. In 1941 Gregg observed a great number of congenital cataracts which he attributed to an epidemic of rubella that had occurred in Australia in 1940. With similar perspicacity, another Australian, McBride (1961), discovered the teratogenic effect of thalidomide.

Until these facts had been established, the general belief of medical investigators was that congenital malformations in man, except those caused by mechanical injuries, were genetically determined.

It is now well recognized that, despite its maternal protection, the development of the mammalian embryo is governed by a constant interplay of hereditary and environmental factors. The genes contain the program for the whole phenotype of the future baby, while the environment supplies the nutrients necessary for growth and differentiation. Hence the expression of the inherited genes depends on exogenous factors which can modify or prevent the development of genetically determined structures, leading to congenital malformations or the death of the embryo.

The reactions of the foetus to environmental factors will be examined here under three headings: the teratogenic principles, the teratogenic agents, and the general mechanisms of teratogenesis.

Teratogenic conditions

The general principles of teratogenesis are not basically different from those underlying deleterious effects in adults. However, the effects of external physical, infectious or chemical agents on the embryo are more complex than in the adult organism. Teratogenesis involves two biological systems: the pregnant female and the embryo. The specific reactions of each can be completely different. So a drug that is non-toxic to the female may still kill the embryo or produce congenital malformations. The problem is complicated by the effects of the placental transfer of drugs and their metabolic fate in the embryo, which are only partly understood. To compete with the various mechanisms which control prenatal development, very complex conditions have to be fulfilled.

The effects of a teratogenic agent on the conceptus depend mainly on (1) the developmental stage, (2) the genetic susceptibility of the embryo and (3) the physiologic or pathologic status of the mother.

The developmental stages

The period in which injurious agents can affect the development of the human embryo is very short. It is largely completed by the 8th week of pregnancy, just about the time a woman first knows that she is pregnant.

During the preimplantation period, when the blastocyst lies free in the uterus and depends for its nutrition on the uterine secretions, exogenous agents can kill the embryo, but there is no evidence that they can produce congenital malformations. This is the period of maximal embryo lethality. However, minor injuries can be survived without obvious harmful consequences to the growing embryo because, during the segmentation stage, many blastomers retain their ability to replace damaged cells by newly formed ones. Once implantation has occurred, at 7-8 days after fertilization, the embryo undergoes rapid and important transformations.

In the sequence of embryonic events, each organ and each system undergoes a critical stage of differentiation at a precise moment in prenatal development. During this critical period the vulnerability of the developing embryo is at its greatest, and specific gross malformations can occur. This is the susceptible period and lasts until the 56th day in man.

The foetal period begins at the end of the 8th week, when little further differentiation of organs remains to be completed. The most important events at this stage are the closure of the palate, the reduction of the umbilical hernia at the end of the 9th week, and the differentiation of the external genitalia at the 12th week. The histogenesis of the central nervous system lasts for the entire period of intrauterine development and is not complete until several months after birth.

Consequently, during the foetal period, teratogenic agents do not cause major morphological malformations but can impair the differentiation of the external genitalia, leading in severe cases to pseudohermaphroditism. Interference with the histogenesis of the central nervous system can lead to various kinds of encephalopathy.

Genetic susceptibility and species differences

The reaction of the embryo to exogenous agents depends on its genetic constitution. It varies not only between different animal species but also within a given species between each strain and even between individuals of the same strain.

Mendelian susceptibility

Hybridization experiments on inbred strains showed that susceptibility to a drug may depend on one or several genes whose effects can be followed through successive generations. It has been established that the susceptibility is not general; the gene action is organ-specific. The tendency to malformation of one organ may depend on several genes, each of which is affected by several teratogens; a strain susceptible to one agent may be found to be resistant to a different teratogen.

These facts indicate that it is not possible to predict the susceptibility of one breed or strain to a compound from its known susceptibility to another compound, however closely chemically related.

Polygenic heredity

This type of heredity is widely represented for a number of characters in man; it is certainly responsible for the susceptibility of a conceptus to different factors constituting the most important process in the multifactorial aetiology of congenital malformations. The results of extensive familial studies suggest that the usual type of malformation depends on a polygenic type of heredity. This shows a transmission which does not fit the mendelian laws. Congenital malformations seem to depend on a continuous specific susceptibility, the small part of the population at one end of the Gaussian curve having malformations. The elegant experiments of Fraser et al. (1957) on the influence of cortisone on the production of cleft palate have demonstrated the mechanism of such action in teratogenic processes.

Physiological or pathological status of the mother

Besides the developmental stage and genetic constitution of the embryo, the other factor affecting the action of a drug is the physiological and pathological condition of the mother. The most important physiological factors are age, diet, hormonal balance and uterine environment. Among pathological conditions, metabolic diseases, diabetes and obesity tend to increase the effects of potentially teratogenic agents.

Teratogenic agents

Physical agents

Radiation

The biological effects of radiation on tissues are well known, although their precise action at a subcellular and molecular level is not yet clear. It is believed that the main lethal effect on cells lies in an alteration of the DNA of the chromosome apparatus. Some of this may be repaired by intracellular recovery processes, with subsequent normal viability of the cell. With increasing doses of radiation, fewer cells maintain their capacity for recovery and division.

It has been shown that X-rays produce a large variety of congenital malformations in various species. In the early stages the anomalies produced are mainly in the central nervous system; at later stages cleft palate and skeletal deformities are observed.

Most of the experimental investigations have been made with high doses, 100 to 200 rads. However Rugh and Grupp (1960) succeeded in producing brain and eye malformations in rodents with doses of 5 to 15 rads. The effects of small doses of radiation are still a matter of discussion. Rugh (1965) stated that to the radiobiologist a small dose would be less than 10 rads. The young human embryo has a very high radiosensitivity between days 18 and 38. After this period higher levels of up to 40 rads are required to produce anomalies. Radiological examination, particularly of the urinary and alimentary system, should be kept to a minimum during pregnancy, and diagnostic radiology of the sacroiliac joints and lumbar spine should be delayed until delivery. Because of the high radiosensitivity of the embryo, it is unwise to use X-ray examination or hysterosalpingography for the diagnosis of early pregnancy. Pregnant women should be submitted to pelvimetry only after a thorough clinical examination.

According to the recommendation of the U.K. Committee on Radiological Hazards, radiological examination for the estimation of foetal maturity should be undertaken only when there is clear need. Multiple pregnancy or breech presentation may properly be established by X-ray examination if the clinical diagnosis is at all doubtful. Other malpresentations and suspected foetal abnormality fully justify X-ray examination, as does suspicion of placenta praevia when accurate clinical diagnosis is not feasible.

The foetus is also very radiosensitive. After the second month of pregnancy the possible induction of leukaemia and other malignant conditions must be considered. Furthermore, exposure of foetuses to doses of a few rads of X-rays can give rise to detectable somatic mutations. Rugh (1958) makes the following comment: 'There are sequelae to foetal irradiations which are not evident for many years even besides the genetic mutations which affect future generations such as the shortening of life, the development of cancer and cataracts, sterility and the increased susceptibility to disease'. The latent period of these cell effects may range from minutes to years.

The danger of radioactivity was tragically confirmed by the atomic bomb explosion. A high incidence of microcephaly and mental retardation has been observed in children whose mothers were close to the hypocenter of the explosion.

There was a close relationship between the incidence of malformations and the gestational age and distance from the hypocenter. Approximately 25% of the survivors had congenital malformations. Furthermore, 64% of the children exposed in utero to the atomic bomb radiation within 1200 meters and who appeared to be normal at birth showed mental retardation at 4.5 years of age. It has also been suggested that prenatal irradiation increases the probability of leukaemia in young children (Stewart, 1957); however, this is still a matter of discussion.

Wood et al. (1967) examined a sample of 1613 Hiroshima and Nagasaki children aged 17 who had been born to mothers exposed to the atomic bomb at a distance of between 2000 and 5000 meters from the hypocenter. In agreement with other reports, they observed limitation of the head circumference and decreased body size. The most prominent effects on growth were seen in the subjects who, in utero, were within 1500 meters of the hypocenter.

The Atomic Bomb Casualty Commission (quoted in Miller, 1969) reported reduced sperm counts and histological gonadal changes in foetal cases in those proximally exposed to the explosion. In women pregnant at the time of the explosion high foetal loss and infant mortality occurred. However, the outcome of pregnancy of women who became pregnant several years after exposure to atomic irradiation was quite normal; there was no congenital malformation and no increase in perinatal or postnatal mortality. Blot and Sawada (1972) examined the fertility of 5000 women over a long period of up to 18 years.

There was no evidence that exposure to high doses of 100 rads of atomic radiation had impaired subsequent fertility, but significant differences were found in the percentage of marriages without conception, depending on contraceptive practice and city of residence.

Hyperthermia

In experimental animals, particularly in rats, hyperthermia produces a high abortion rate. A few of the survivors had eye and teeth deformities (McFarlane et al., 1957). Focal hyperthermia in the uterus causes central nervous system and eye anomalies.

Edwards et al. (1971) showed that in mice and guinea pigs hyperthermia produced abortions, brain anomalies and impaired histogenesis of the central nervous system.

In guinea pigs the brain weight was reduced by 8% when the maternal body temperature was raised to 41.5°C between days 20 and 23.

Infectious agents

Rubella

Gregg (1941) demonstrated that rubella occurring in early pregnancy could lead to abortion or to a typical syndrome of ocular, cardiovascular and mental defects. The first epidemiological surveys suggested that rubella contracted during the first trimester of pregnancy resulted in foetal damage in approximatively 70-80% of cases. Prospective studies established that the risk was smaller than that. Rubella infection in the first 4 weeks is likely to harm 60% of embryos; in weeks 5-8 the frequency of malformations is 26%; and in weeks 9-12 it falls to 8%.

Rubella embryopathies represent only a small percentage of the total incidence of congenital malformations. However, in the epidemic in New York in 1964, 1% of pregnancies became rubella casualties and approximatively 20,000 children developed birth defects associated with rubella.

The rubella virus reaches the embryo through the maternal circulation and persists through pregnancy and for several months after birth. In certain lesions, such as a cataractous lens, the virus can still be found after months or even years.

Rubella vaccination has completely changed the potential danger of this disease. It has been suggested that all children between the age of one year and puberty should be immunized against rubella in order to eliminate the disease. According to Krugman and Katz (1974), in the last 5 years more than 55 million doses of rubella vaccine have been distributed. They were used for routine immunization of children between 1 and 12 years of age and for selective immunization of susceptible women of childbearing age. Use of the vaccine is believed to have protected about 10,000 and perhaps even 20,000 pregnancies either from abortion or from the dysmorphogenetic effect of intrauterine rubella infection. The incidence of arthralgia and neuromuscular disorders has been considerably reduced by improving the preparation of the vaccine.

The problem of communicability has been solved. It has been shown that immunized children are not contagious. Consequently, pregnancy, which is a contraindication to vaccination of the mother, is an indication for vaccination of her child, because an immunized susceptible child may introduce wild rubella into the home.

The risk of rubella vaccination to the foetus has not been definitely assessed, but it has been proved that viraemia does not occur after reinfection. Therefore it is unlikely that foetal infection will occur in association with reinfection after either vaccination or the natural disease.

Cytomegalic inclusion disease

The characteristic feature of this disease is the presence of enlarged cells with inclusion bodies separated from the nuclear membrane by a light halo. The inclusions are abundant in the salivary glands and to a lesser extent in the viscera.

It is assumed that only prenatal or neonatal viral infections lead to serious accidents, including postnatal death. In pregnant women the viraemia is transmitted to the chorionic villi and to various embryonic tissues. Early infection leads to abortion and congenital malformations. The clinical picture involved hepatosplenomegaly, jaundice, thrombocytopenic purpura, anaemia, intrauterine growth retardation, microcephaly and paraventricular calcification of the skull.

Herpes virus

Schaeffer (1965) claims that genital herpes can cause congenital malformations similar to those produced by cytomegalic inclusion disease. In several cases from which herpes virus type 2 was isolated a large variety of malformations was observed, e.g. microcephaly, intracranial calcifications and various eye malformations including microphthalmia and retinal dysplasia.

Toxoplasmosis

A large variety of severe congenital malformations can be produced by prenatal infection with *Toxoplasma gondii*. The most frequent anomalies are microcephaly, hydrocephaly, calcification, microphthalmia, chorioretinitis and functional disturbances of the brain.

Most of the infections are subclinical. The diagnosis of toxoplasmosis requires laboratory tests for confirmation.

The frequency of maternal toxoplasmosis during pregnancy is about 8 per 1000. Of 47 infants born to mothers who acquired the infection during pregnancy 4 died in the neonatal period with generalized toxoplasmosis; 3 were living with sequelae; 13 were infected without sequelae; and 27 escaped infection (Desmonts et al., 1965).

Chemical agents

A large variety of chemical agents, including drugs, are capable of producing malformations in experimental animals and in man. We will examine only a few drugs which are likely to be frequently used in pregnant women as steroidal hormones, psycho-active drugs, antiemetics, analgesics, hypoglycaemic agents, antitumour drugs and disinfectants.

Sex steroids

Testosterone and its analogues have a masculinizing effect in female foetuses. In girls masculinization of the urogenital sinus takes the form of hypertrophy of the clitoris and atrophy of the labia. If the drug is given before the 12th week of pregnancy complete fusion of the labia may occur. Since Wilkins (1969) reported the first case, a further 100 or more cases of masculinization of female foetuses associated with the use of 17α-ethinyltestosterone and 17α-ethinyl-19-nortestosterone have been described to date.

The female sex hormones, progesterone and oestradiol, are considered to have no adverse effects on the embryo.

Diethylstilboestrol, a potent synthetic oestrogen, has a feminizing effect on male rat foetuses. Herbst et al. (1971) reported that adenocarcinoma of the vagina occurred in relatively young girls whose mothers received stilboestrol treatment during the first trimester of pregnancy. The causal relationship between stilboestrol therapy of the mothers and vaginal cancer in the daughters, although not completely demonstrated, seems highly probable.

Herbst et al. (1972) found a high proportion of vaginal adenosis in girls of 13-14 years exposed to diethylstilboestrol in utero. The exposure was before the 12th week of pregnancy and the usual dosage was 10 mg per day.

Clear-cell adenocarcinoma of the cervix after maternal treatment with stilboestrol was also reported by Noller et al. (1972).

Clomiphene, an ovulation-inducing drug, certainly has a teratogenic potential in animals. Eneroth et al. (1971) observed hydramnios and cataracts in rats when the drug was given from day 6 to day 14. However, in primates, Courtney and Valerio (1968) did not observe malformations with doses of 1 to 3 mg/kg during the critical stages of embryogenesis. In human subjects this drug increases the frequency of multiple pregnancies but there is no evidence that the incidence of congenital malformations is higher when the mothers have been treated with it.

Contraceptive steroids

In animal experiments Tuchmann-Duplessis and Mercier-Parot (1972) have examined the effect of a contraceptive steroid, Enidrel (norethynodrel with mestranol), on the pituitary hypothalamic system and on prenatal and perinatal development. Even with high doses, no congenital malformations were produced, and there was no impairment of postnatal development. In human subjects no mutagenic effects or increase in chromosomal aberrations were observed in women who conceived during contraceptive treatment or several months after withdrawal of the drug. In agreement with experimental results, clinical data indicate that contraceptive drugs have no masculinizing effects.

The teratogenic danger which has been suspected for some time has not been substantiated, though a very large series of clinical observations have been made. In a prospective study sponsored by the French Ministry of Health Spira et al. (1972) compared 9,566 women who took sex hormones or contraceptive drugs with 8387 control women given no treatment. The patients were followed up from the first trimester of pregnancy to delivery and the children were examined at birth and several months later. Whether the women took oestrogens, progesterone compounds or a combination of both, the incidence of congenital malformations was no different.

Recently there have been several claims of a possible teratogenic effect of sex hormones. Janerich et al. (1974) made a retrospective study of 108 mothers who gave birth to infants with congenital reduction deformities of the limbs born in New York in 1968-1973 and compared them to controls matched for race and maternal age. Morphological defects were defined as the absence of an arm or leg or part thereof, including fingers or toes.

A total of 15 mothers claimed to have taken steroid hormones during pregnancy, as compared with 4 control mothers. Six had break-through pregnancies while on the pill and 6 others were given steroids as a 'supportive measure'. Three took pregnancy test drugs while pregnant. In each control group there was only one case for each similar category. All the affected children whose mothers took sex steroids were male. Two of the six pregnancies associated with a history of pill failure resulted in twins; only one of each pair was deformed.

Janerich et al. think that there could be a causal relationship between the sex steroid therapy and the limb defects. However, they also consider the possibility of an association with some underlying maternal disorder. In that case the hormones effectively supported an abnormal pregnancy which would otherwise have been aborted.

Sex steroids have also been incriminated in the aetiology of heart and vascular malformations. Levy et al. (1973) noted a high incidence of hormone treatment in pregnancies which resulted in the birth of infants with transposition of the great vessels. Of 76 mothers interviewed 10 gave a history of hormone treatment in the first trimester. Nora and Nora (1974) reported the use of progestagen or oestrogen in 20 of 224 cases of heart disease, compared with 4 of 262 controls.

Harlap et al. (1975) examined 11,468 babies of whom 432 (3.8%) were born after definite or probable administration of oestrogens or progesterones to the mother. They found that the risk of major malformations was about 26% higher in those exposed or probably exposed to hormones than in those with no history of exposure, whereas for minor malformations the increased risk was about 33%.

The significance of these studies is still uncertain. An Editorial in the *Lancet* (1974) said that if there is a link between the various malformations and hormone ingestion during early pregnancy, this teratogenic effect 'is remarkably non-specific'.

Corticosteroids

Cortisone produces cleft palates and various cardiac abnormalities in mice and rabbits. Hydrocortisone and ACTH have similar effects in mice. The incidence of malformations varies according to the dose of cortisone and the strain of the animal that is being studied.

We are still assessing the susceptibility of the human foetus to cortisone. Several cases of cleft palate have been observed in infants born to mothers treated with cortisone during pregnancy. Popert (1962) analysed several hundred cases found in the literature, and discovered that 1% of children exposed to cortisone in utero had cleft palates. This incidence is slightly higher than in a random sample and Popert therefore considers cortisone to be a weak teratogen in man. However, taking into account the fact that cortisone is only administered to women who have a pathological condition, one must be cautious about making any definite statement relating the cleft palates that have been observed with cortisone therapy. Although the risk of giving cortisone seems to be slight, it is wiser to administer it to pregnant women only if the medical condition really justifies taking the risk.

Warrel and Taylor (1968) examined the outcome of 43 pregnancies in prednisolone-treated patients and found 8 stillbirths and 9 foetuses judged to have been at risk during pregnancy or parturition. Compared to a similar control group, there was an excess of harmful effects. Although this observation suggests a very high risk to the foetus from corticosteroid therapy during pregnancy, Scott (1968) considers that if the same category of patients had had no corticosteroid therapy the outcome of pregnancy might have been worse.

Oral hypoglycaemic drugs

Several hypoglycaemic sulphonamides (carbutamide, tolbutamide and dimethylbiguanide) are teratogenic in rodents. In most cases the abnormalities are observed in the eye and the central nervous system, yet skeletal abnormalities, cleft palate and even shortening of the maxilla can be produced (Tuchmann-Duplessis and Mercier-Parot, 1963a). The teratogenic action does not seem to be related to the chemical structure of the compound nor to its specific pharmacological properties.

Abortions and malformations in man have been attributed to the use of hypoglycaemic agents. No definite conclusions can be drawn, however, since the available clinical data indicates that both normal and abnormal children can be born to mothers who have received copious amounts in early pregnancy. Until there is more information on the subject, oral hypoglycaemic agents should be considered to be less safe than insulin and therefore should be avoided in treatment of pregnant women.

Recent reports (Sutherland et al., 1973) suggest that chlorpropamide in daily doses of 200 mg is harmless to the foetus. The use of this drug is best confined to women with mild diabetes in whom good control can be attained with doses of 200 mg. Foetal death has been observed in badly controlled pregnancies where doses of 500 mg had been given. Jackson (1974) made similar observations and stressed that in pregnant women the diabetic state should not be controlled with doses exceeding 250 mg daily.

A high perinatal mortality was observed after the use of 500 mg chlorpropamide; no congenital malformations were observed. Notelovitz (1974) considers that hypoglycaemic biguanides do not constitute an increased risk to the foetus. However, he thinks that they should not be used in early pregnancy.

Hyperglycaemic agents

Experiments on alloxan diabetes in mice have repeatedly shown malformations. Glucagon is teratogenic in rats. By injecting 300-600 μg we were able to produce various eye malformations ranging from glaucoma to microphthalmia. Other hyperglycaemic agents, such as galactose-2-desoxyglucose and fluroacetate, are also teratogenic in rats (De Meyer, 1961).

Cholesterolaemic agents

The frequent association of diabetes and disorders of lipid metabolism led us to examine the action of Triton WR-1339 (tyloxapol), which causes hyperlipaemia and a significant rise in total body cholesterol. Large doses of Triton WR-1339 cause a high percentage of abortions and 15-20% gross malformations in rodents. These results suggest that the various fertility disorders observed in diabetics may be related not only to their hyperglycaemia but also to other metabolic disorders (Tuchmann-Duplessis and Mercier-Parot, 1964b). A hypocholesterolaemic agent, triparanol (MER-29), produces multiple malformations of the central nervous system in rats and mice (Roux and Dupuis, 1961).

Psycho-active drugs

Several of these have been incriminated as the cause of human malformations following clinical and experimental demonstration of the teratogenic action of thalidomide.

Glutarimides We investigated two chemically related compounds of thalidomide, 2-ethyl-2-phenyl-glutarimide (Doriden) and phenglutarimide (Aturbane), which had become suspect. No malformations could be observed even with very high doses, including those toxic to the mother (Tuchmann-Duplessis and Mercier-Parot, 1963b, 1964a). This example demonstrates how chemical structure, pharmacological properties and teratogenic action are all independent of one another.

Phenothiazines A large number of phenothiazines have been used for long periods in pregnancy to relieve tension and nausea. Although in a few isolated cases a slight teratogenic action of chlorpromazine and prochlorpemazine has been reported in rats, there has been no proof of any toxic effect on a human foetus even when the drug had been taken for several months.

Benzodiazepines Several compounds of this group, such as chlordiazepoxide (Librium), diazepam (Valium) and nitrazepam (Mogadon) are widely used in clinical practice. Experimental investigations in rats and rabbits did not reveal any teratogenic effects. Neither the progress of pregnancy nor the development of the offspring were affected, even when doses 20 to 40 times higher than the therapeutic dosage were used.

It has been claimed that benzodiazepines cause chromosomal aberrations, but detailed in vitro and in vivo studies did not confirm this. The clinical data suggest that, although the benzodiazepines rapidly cross the placenta, they have no adverse effects on the offspring.

Diazepam, which has been used for some time in cases of threatened abortion, does not seem to increase the normal rate of congenital malformation. According to Wallner et al. (1973) no significant difference in anomalies has been observed between women treated for threatened abortion with sex hormones and those treated with a combination of sex hormones and diazepam.

However, Istvan (1970) reported the case of a child born without thumbs and a congenital dislocation of the head of the right radius. The mother had received 6 mg diazepam daily in the first trimester of pregnancy, but the possible connections between these malformations and the ingested drug is doubtful.

The available experimental and clinical data suggest that neither chlordiazepoxide nor diazepam have a teratogenic potential.

Recently Milkovich and Van den Berg (1974) claimed that there might be an association between the use of chlordiazepoxide (and another tranquilizer, meprobamate) in early pregnancy and an increased incidence of severe congenital malformations. This assumption was based on a prospective epidemiological study that included 19,044 live births. The rate of anomalies was four times higher in infants born to mothers who took this drug than in those born to mothers who did not. The heterogeneity of the malformations found in these children and the lack of similar findings in other epidemiological studies led us to doubt that the two drugs were potential human teratogens (Tuchmann-Duplessis, 1975).

In an independent follow-up study, Hartz et al. (1975) compared 1870 children exposed to meprobamate or chlordiazepoxide in the first trimester or at other times during pregnancy with 48,412 children who were not. They concluded that there was no evidence that either of these drugs were teratogenic. No relationship with major malformations, cardiac anomalies or stillbirths was found. In addition, as judged by mental and motor scores at the ages of 8 months and 4 years, there was no evidence that these drugs caused brain damage.

Butyrophenones Large doses of haloperidol can delay implantation in rats and in mice. In our experience this action is due to a modification of the gonadotropic activity of the maternal pituitary, leading to excessive release of luteotrophic hormone.

Reserpine, which is used in hypertension and in psychiatric disorders, may affect the foetus. A syndrome characterized by lethargy, bradycardia, hypothermia and nasal congestion has been described. A similar syndrome due to depletion of catecholamine stores has been produced in guinea pigs, but no abnormalities were observed.

Hallucinogens The influence of hallucinogens, particularly of lysergic acid diethylamide (LSD), has raised great interest in recent years. A large number of studies and case reports have been published incriminating LSD as a chromosome-breaking agent, a mutagen or a teratogen in experimental animals and in man. There is evidence that LSD crosses the placenta and enters the foetus at different stages of gestation, as seen from studies on ^{14}C-labeled LSD in mice and hamsters (Idanpään-Heikkila and Schoolar, 1969).

Studies of selected groups of hospitalized psychiatric patients who had taken LSD and other drugs previously yielded contradictory results. Zellweger et al. (1967) and Nielsen et al. (1969) attributed a variety of malformations observed in neonates to their parents' use of LSD. Berlin and Jacobson (1970), in a series of 112 women who had taken LSD before and during pregnancy, observed an increased rate of malformations and abortions.

These data concerned users of illicit LSD. The problem is quite different where pure LSD is concerned (Judd et al., 1969). The positive results are proba-bly related to the general effects of drug abuse, involving a combination of other factors such as frequent viral infections and physical debility in drug users. From studies performed by several research teams (Tjio et al., 1969; Dishotsky et al., 1971; Long, 1972), it can be concluded that 'pure LSD ingested in moderate doses does not produce chromosome damage... and is not teratogenic in man' (Dishotsky et al., 1971). The postulated mutagenic action of LSD has not been substantiated.

Anticonvulsants   Diphenylhydantoin, a drug frequently used in pregnant epileptics rapidly crosses the placenta. High concentrations are attained in the foetal liver and in the brain one hour after intravenous injection into the mother. In rats, the ratio of foetal to maternal concentrations of diphenylhydantoin is approximately 2:1 in favour of the foetus. Growth retardation and a large variety of congenital malformations can be produced in mice and rats by diphen-ylhydantoin (Gibson and Becker, 1968; Harbison and Becker, 1969, 1972; Tuch-mann-Duplessis and Mercier-Parot, 1973; Mercier-Parot and Tuchmann-Duplessis, 1974).

Various drugs used in epilepsy have been suspected to have adverse effects on the human embryo. Meadow (1970) found a high incidence of facial and heart malformations in children born to treated epileptic mothers. The most common defects noticed were cleft lips and palates, sometimes associated with cardiac defects. Speidel and Meadow (1972), in a retrospective survey of 427 preg-nancies in 186 epileptic women, showed that congenital malformations were more common in the children of epileptic women taking anticonvulsant drugs than in the general population.

Besides congenital anomalies, mental subnormality occurred in 1.5% of the epileptic mothers' children, compared with 0.2% in a control group. The perina-tal mortality rate was 42.5 per 1000 for pregnancies in which anticonvulsants were taken; this was nearly twice the regional rate. The rate for all epileptic women was 28.6 per 1000. The increased perinatal mortality was mainly due to congenital malformations and to spontaneous haemorrhage, which occurred in 6 out of 388 births.

A survey of congenital malformations in infants born to mothers in Cardiff over a seven-year-period revealed a malformation rate of 2.7%. Where the mother had a history of epilepsy and had been on anticonvulsants during the first trimester the rate was 6.7% (Lowe, 1973).

Stimulants of the central nervous system Among drugs used as psycholeptics, MAO-inhibitors and amitriptyline derivatives have been investigated.

Nialamide, a well known MAO-inhibitor, is not teratogenic. We investigated its influence on pregnancy in the rat (Tuchmann-Duplessis and Mercier-Parot, 1962). High doses given immediately after fertilisation or after implantation cause foetal resorption but no congenital malformations.

Dexamphetamine sulphate is teratogenic in A/Jax mice (Nora et al., 1965). Large doses administered parenterally at the onset of pregnancy caused foetal resorption, retarded growth and malformations. 11% of the offspring had anophthalmia or microphthalmia, and 18% had palatoschisis. In rabbits no teratogenic effects were observed.

This drug has been incriminated in the aetiology of human malformations. Clinical data suggest the possibility of a teratogenic risk. Nora et al. (1970), in a study of 184 mothers of infants with heart malformations, found a higher incidence of amphetamine ingestion than in a control group. Levin (1971) found a high incidence of biliary tract atresia among the offspring of mothers taking amphetamines.

One of the analogues of this drug, methamphetamine hydrochloride, when given at a dose of 10 mg/kg causes 13% gross malformations in mice. In rabbits even small doses of 1.5 mg/kg administered between days 12-15 or between days 15-20 have a teratogenic effect. Approximatively 15% of the survivors have gross congenital malformations (Kasirsky and Tansy, 1971).

Imipramine has been suspected of causing human malformations in some circumstances. It has been claimed that when this antidepressant is taken in early pregnancy it can harm morphogenesis, leading to various malformations of the central nervous system and of the limbs (McBride, 1972). A few experimental data seem to substantiate this hypothesis. Robson and Sullivan (1963) used high doses of imipramine to induce various malformations of the central nervous system in rabbits. However, we did not observe malformations in rabbits or mice even though large doses of imipramine were administered throughout pregnancy.

Careful epidemiological studies carried out recently have led to a more optimistic evaluation of this drug. Crombie et al. (1972) analysed the outcome of 19 cases in which imipramine was administered during the early weeks of pregnancy. No abnormalities in this group were reported at birth or subsequently. In another group in which 28 prescriptions for amitriptyline were given, the outcome of pregnancy was normal. Kuenssberg and Knox (1972) reviewed 15,000 pregnancies in Scotland. There were 17 mothers for whom imipramine was prescribed within the first 10 weeks of pregnancy. No abnormalities were reported in the 14 children. One mother aborted and 2 gave birth to malformed children. One had defective abdominal muscles and a possible abnormality of the gut; the other had a diaphragmatic hernia. Of 31 mothers for whom amitriptyline was prescribed, 28 had normal babies. One aborted; there was one stillbirth, and one child was born with hypospadias. This study suggests that these antidepressants are not associated with a high teratogenic risk.

In animals conflicting results have been reported with lithium. It is generally believed to have a very low teratogenic potential.

The number of patients with recurrent manic-depressive disorders treated with lithium carbonate is increasing constantly, and a high number of pregnant women have experienced this treatment. Schou et al. (1973) made a retrospective investigation of 118 children born to mothers who were given lithium during the first trimester of pregnancy. They concluded that the risk of teratogenic effects is lower than one might expect from certain experimental data. However, they still could not answer the question of whether or not lithium is teratogenic in man.

Analgesics   Salicylates rapidly cross the placental barrier. In the mouse, the drug can be found in the foetus 5 minutes after administration to the mother. The salicylate compounds are hydrolyzed to salicyclic acid and thereafter transformed to acid and phenolic glucuronides. A small proportion of salicylic acid is hydroxylated to gentisic acid.

Warnaky and Takacs (1959) demonstrated that very high doses of methyl or sodium salicylate (300 to 600 mg/kg body weight) are teratogenic in the rat. A large variety of malformations of the central nervous system, the skeleton and the viscera, including cardiovascular defects, were observed.

In *Macaca mulatta* daily doses of 300 mg/kg of acetylsalicylic acid resulted in either abortion or maternal death (Tanimura, 1972). In the rhesus monkey doses of 400-500 mg/kg of acetylsalicylic acid administered between days 18 and 24 of pregnancy are embryotoxic but only occasionally teratogenic (Wilson, 1971).

The question whether salicylates in therapeutic doses cause human malformations is not yet solved and will require large-scale prospective studies. Meanwhile it seems prudent not to use heavy doses of salicylates in pregnant women.

The administration of aspirin during the second part of gestation can prolong the duration of gestation and parturition. Tuchmann-Duplessis et al. (1974) have shown that in rats doses of 200 mg/kg of aspirin given between day 15 of gestation and delivery, or only 2 days before delivery, cause prolongation of the gestation time and of the duration of parturition in the majority of animals.

Lewis and Schulman (1973) concluded from an epidemiological retrospective study that in women taking more than 3.25 g aspirin in the last trimester of pregnancy, there was a prolongation of the gestation period and of labour.

Collins and Turner (1973) concluded from a prospective study that in women regularly taking aspirin a high proportion have a prolonged gestation period (16% as compared to 2% in a control group). Parturition accidents, post-natal bleeding and delivery retardation ending in caesarian operation were 7 times more frequent than normal.

Other analgesics, such as morphine, meperidine, scopolamine and chloral hydrate, which all cross the placenta, are not teratogenic. If administered in the last months of pregnancy, however, morphine does have a definite depressant action on the foetus. In mothers addicted to morphine the foetus can develop a syndrome of physiological dependence. In such rare cases a withdrawal syndrome has been observed in the newborn.

Anticoagulants

Two groups of anticoagulants are available: heparin, which does not cross the placenta, and the coumarine derivatives of low molecular weight, which easily enter the foetal circulation.

Although bishydroxycoumarin (dicoumarol) and its analogues are nearly completely bound to plasma proteins, they enter the foetal compartment and exert a more pronounced anticoagulative effect on the foetus than on the mother.

The toxic effects of bishydroxycoumarin might also be attributable to the enzymatic immaturity of the foetal liver. The detoxification mechanism, which includes conjugation with glucuronic acid, is deficient and even minute quantities of free bishydroxycoumarin can interfere with prothrombin synthesis in the liver. A further complication of coumarin therapy may occur when the mother simultaneously receives barbiturates. It has been well demonstrated that in adults phenobarbital decreases the action of other drugs by increasing the rate at which they are metabolized to pharmacologically inactive compounds.

Oral anticoagulants have been suspected of producing foetal morbidity and mortality as well as bone malformations (Kerber et al., 1968). However, this has not been substantiated. The effect of early oral anticoagulant treatment is still uncertain, but in several cases reported and in personal observations in 5 patients treated before conception and during the first trimester the outcome of pregnancy was normal.

Hirsch et al. (1970) treated 15 pregnant women with heparin and 10 with warfarin. The mean length of therapy was 4-5 weeks with heparin and 14 weeks with warfarin. There were 3 minor haemorrhagic episodes during anticoagulant therapy. No foetal or neonatal complications occurred. Taking into consideration their own experience and the results of various case reports, the authors concluded that oral anticoagulants do not increase the risk of foetal damage unless continued until term.

Despite the theoretical risk, there is no evidence that anticoagulants in therapeutic doses increase the incidence of maternal haemorrhage before, during or after delivery.

Antitumour drugs

A great number of anticancer chemotherapeutic agents belonging to various chemical groups have been investigated. Most of them are toxic; they cause hypoplasia of the bone marrow and have an inhibitory effect on epithelial proliferation.

Embryonic cells are much more sensitive to the toxic effects of antitumour drugs than adult cells. Therefore most compounds have deleterious actions on the embryo at lower doses than in the adult. They are embryotoxic and frequently also teratogenic.

While in experimental animals a very large number of compounds induce congenital malformations, the teratogenic potential in man has only been demonstrated for aminopterin, methotrexate, busulphan, cyclophosphamide and chlorambucil.

Antibiotics

Most antibiotics, such as penicillin, streptomycin, dehydrostreptomycin, tetracycline, oxytetracycline and oxymethyl-penicillin, cross the placental barrier rapidly and are found at high levels in the embryo and in the amniotic fluid. After extensive use the impression gained is that most antibiotics are harmless to the human embryo. Drugs such as rifamycin and puromycin, which act on cell enzymatic activities, disturb protein synthesis.

Rifamycin, a highly active antituberculous drug given in large doses (150 mg/kg) can induce congenital malformations in rats and mice. The most frequent malformations are spina bifida and cleft palate. In the rabbit no congenital anomalies were found (Tuchmann-Duplessis and Mercier-Parot, 1969).

The clinical data suggest that the potential danger of rifamycin for the human foetus is limited. From a retrospective study in 313 tuberculous women who had received rifamycin and/or ethambutol during pregnancy, Jentgens (1973) concluded that both drugs are devoid of embryotoxic or teratogenic effects. However, in this epidemiological study there were only 38 women treated at conception or during the first trimester of pregnancy. Therefore it is still unwise to draw definite conclusions.

Rubidomycin (daunorubicin), an antibiotic used in antitumour therapy, has been found to be teratogenic in rats. With doses ranging from 1 to 3 mg/kg, Roux and Taillemite (1969) observed a high percentage of eye and visceral malformations. Julou et al. (1967) could not produce malformations in rats or mice.

In man, the antibiotics routinely used may be considered to be fairly safe for the embryo. Ravid and Toaff (1972) made a prospective study of 100 women who were given antibiotic treatment throughout pregnancy and an untreated control group of 911 mothers. There was no difference in these two groups in the incidence of congenital malformations. The malformations found among the children of the treated group were of the same morphological type as those found in a normal healthy population and could not be attributed to the antibiotic treatment of the mothers. The authors concluded: 'The assumption that antibiotic treatment in early pregnancy contributed to the genesis of congenital defects seems rather unlikely. Antibiotic therapy should therefore not be withheld during pregnancy if otherwise indicated.'

Sulphonamides

Most sulphonamides reach the same blood concentration in the foetus as in the maternal circulation within 1 or 2 hours. Long-acting compounds, such as sulphapyridine, sulphasoxazole, sulphacetamide, sulphadiazine, sulphathiazole, and sulphamerazine, can produce congenital malformations in rats.

Sulphonamides may bring about an increase in the incidence of kernicterus, since they cause penetration of unconjugated bilirubin into the central nervous tissue. Similar adverse effects have not been shown to occur in the foetus.

Mechanisms

A large variety of mechanisms can be implicated in the teratogenic action of chemical and other environmental agents. Theoretically, it is possible for the agent to act directly or indirectly on the embryo or foetus, by modifying the maternal metabolism.

Direct action on the foetus is possible since many chemicals given to the pregnant animals, such as some antibiotics, sulphonamides and thalidomide, reach the embryo without being modified.

It is perhaps through indirect action on the endocrine balance of the foetus that compounds such as steroid hormones can induce virilisation of human foetuses. Modification of the foeto-placental unit by biogenic amines can produce malformations by reducing placental transfer. Modification of foetal nutrition can be suspected in the case of certain chemicals such as trypan blue.

The particulated dye is retained in the visceral yolk-sac endoderm, which plays a very important role in nutrition of the embryo.

The possibility that inhibition of embryotrophic nutrition may produce congenital malformations could also apply to other compounds that may act as inhibitors of constituent enzymes of the foetal membranes.

Drugs that modify maternal and possibly foetal metabolism, such as hypoglycaemic or hypolipidaemic agents or compounds which affect lysosomal mechanisms, frequently cause congenital malformations. Consequently, it has been suggested that such anomalies are connected with failure, or lack of production, of a basic cell constituent.

Malformations may further be associated with the production of an abnormal cell constituent, a protein or nucleotide. As suggested by Chaube and Murphy (1968), antimetabolites may induce malformations by competitive action on nucleic acid metabolism. By this effect they may modify specific protein synthesis and act in a way comparable to genetic factors.

Another factor involving maternal reactions may originate from metabolic interactions between various drugs, pesticides, food additives and a variety of environmental chemicals. These effects are due to the activity of microsomal enzymes, particularly of the liver, that may be stimulated or inhibited by chemicals metabolized on the cytoplasmic membranes. In this way, substances foreign to the body may modify the metabolism of other chemicals that are administered at the same time.

Whatever the general mechanism of the noxious effect on the conceptus, the teratogenic action results finally in an impairment of the normal processes of development, and the final result depends principally on the susceptibility of the animal, which is extremely variable. Some species are highly resistant to one factor and sensitive to an other; different strains in the same species are widely different in their susceptibility and even in the same litter some embryos may be quite normal while others are dead or show malformations.

This can be explained, at least in part, by genetical differences and the time involved in the particular type of interaction. The latter may be critical because of the strictly programmed sequence of intertissue reactions resulting in differentiation, and also because of the different susceptibility of the various phases of growth in the cell populations.

The influence of genetic susceptibility, which has been explored using pure animal strains, has already been discussed.

Cell kinetics

The effect of a teratogenic agent may depend on the precise phase of multiplication of a tissue. A number of teratogenic agents are known to interfere directly with cell multiplication. Recent progress in cell kinetics has provided new insight into the mechanisms of this action on the cell cycle. A great amount of precise data has been obtained through the study of tumour cell multiplication and of the action of different drugs which impair this multiplication. These studies afford a model which can be used in embryology. Impairment of the multiplication of populations of cells in a developing organ results in a malformation.

These substances may be classified into: cycle-specific agents, which act on any cell in its generation cycle; and phase-specific agents, which act very specifically on one phase of the cell cycle. For instance, a compound specific for the S-phase will act only on those cells which happen to be present in the S-phase at the time the agent is present.

The teratogenic action depends again on a threshold effect determined by the number of cells entering the sensitive phase during the time the teratogen is present. If the agent intervenes at the beginning of a multiplication wave at one stage of organogenesis, it is easy to imagine how a very small difference in the beginning of the wave in embryos of the same litter may modify the cytostatic effects of the antiproliferative agent. This offers wide possibilities for experimentation. Some interesting information is already available on the kinetics of embryonic cells. Köhler (1970) showed that the speed of the generation cycle of embryonic cells in the rat varies considerably and rapidly in the course of embryonic life. Between days 11 and 12 the embryonic cells grow exponentially, the duration of the whole cycle being 8 hours (3 cell generations in 24 hours). During this period the G1 phase is probably missing, most cells being in the G2 and late S-phase. These modalities of cell kinetics change from one day to the next. Such data are a valuable aid in understanding the great differences that may be shown by embryos of the same litter, and therefore of similar genetic background, that are exposed to the same environment through the same maternal organism.

Conclusions

The thalidomide accidents led to overemphasis on the potential danger to the foetus from drugs taken by the mother. The experience gained in recent years has led to a less pessimistic view of the teratogenic danger of drugs. It is now understood that very complex conditions have to be fulfilled before there is a threat to the basic mechanism which controls prenatal development. To produce a congenital malformation not only must the teratogenic agent be given in an appropriate dosage and at a very precise stage of morphogenesis, but the embryo must also have genetic susceptibility to the agent.

Hybridization experiments in inbred strains showed that susceptibility to a drug may depend on one or several genes, the effects of which can be followed through successive generations. The susceptibility is not general; the gene action is organ-specific. An organ's tendency to malformation may depend on several genes, each being affected by various teratogens; a strain susceptible to one agent may be found to be resistant if a different teratogen is used. These facts indicate that it is not possible to predict the susceptibility of one breed or strain to a compound from its known susceptibility to another chemically related compound.

The potential action of environmental factors during intrauterine life is of particular concern because of its irreversible nature. A large variety of teratogenic agents have been discovered in animals through well designed experiments. Fortunately, such a complex sequence of events only exceptionally occurs spontaneously, so only a very limited number of these agents have been proved to be teratogenic in man.

While the evaluation of the teratogenic risk in pregnant women has to be made with particular caution, excessive fear should not lead one to deprive women of the benefits of efficient drugs.

The prospects for the detection of environmental teratogenic agents are favourable. As more experience is gained through experimental investigations and human epidemiological studies, preventive measures should become a possibility.

References

Berlin, C. M. and Jacobson, C. B. (1970): *Pediat. Res., 4,* 377 (abstract).
Blot, W. J. and Sawada, H. (1972): *Amer. J. hum. genet., 24,* 613.
Chaube, S. and Murphy, M. L. (1968): In: *Advances in Teratology, 3,* 181. Logos Press, London.
Collins, E. and Turner, G. (1973): *Lancet, 2,* 1494.
Courtney, K. D. and Valerio, D. A. (1968): *Teratology, 1,* 163.
Crombie, D. L., Pinsent, R. F. H. and Fleming, D. (1972): *Brit. med. J., 1,* 745.
De Meyer, R. (1961): *Etude Expérimentale de la Glycorégulation Gravidique et de l'Action Tératogène des Perturbations du Métabolisme Glucidique.* Arscia, Brussels.
Desmonts, G., Couvreur, J. and Rachid, M. S. (1965): *Arch. franç. Pédiat., 22,* 1183.
Dishotsky, N. I., Loughman, W. D., Mogar, R. E. and Lipscomb, W. R. (1971): *Science, 172,* 43.
Edwards, M. J. (1969): *Teratology, 2,* 313.
Edwards, M. J., Penny, R. H. C., and Zevnik, I. (1971): *Brain Res., 28,* 341.
Eneroth, G., Eneroth, V., Forsberg, U., Grant, C. A. and Gustafsson, J. A. (1971): *Teratology, 4,* 487.
Fraser, F. C., Walker, B. E. and Trasler, D. G. (1957): *Pediatrics, 19,* 782.

Gibson, J. E. and Becker, B. A. (1968): *Proc. Soc. exp. Biol. (N. Y.), 128,* 905.
Gregg, N. (1941): *Trans. ophthal. Soc. Aust., 3,* 35.
Harbison, R. D. and Becker, B. A. (1969): *Teratology, 2,* 305.
Harbison, R. D. and Becker, B. A. (1972): *Toxicol. appl. Pharmacol., 22,* 193.
Harlap, S., Prywes, R. and Davies, A. M. (1975): *Lancet, 1,* 682.
Hartz, S. C., Heinonen, O. P., Shapiro, S., Siskind, V. and Slone, D. (1975): *New Engl. J. Med., 292,* 727.
Herbst, A. L., Ulfelder, H. and Poskanzer, D. C. (1971): *New Engl. J. Med., 284,* 878.
Herbst, A. L., Kurman, R. J. and Scully, R. E. (1972): *Obstet. and Gynec., 40,* 287.
Hirsh, J., Cade, J. F. and O'Sullivan, E. F. (1970): *Brit. med. J., 1,* 270.
Idanpään-Heikkila, J. E. and Schoolar, J. C. (1969): *Lancet, 2,* 221.
Istvan, E. J. (1970): *Canad. med. Ass. J., 103,* 1394.
Jackson, W. P. (1974): *Lancet, 2,* 843.
Janerich, D. I., Piper, J. M. and Glebatis, D. M. (1974): *New Engl. J. Med., 291,* 697.
Jentgens, H. (1973): *Praxis Pneumol., 27,* 479.
Judd, L. L., Brandkamp, W. W. and McGlothlin, W. H. (1969): *Amer. J. Psychiat., 126,* 626.
Julou, L., Ducrot, R., Fournel, J., Gauter, P., Maral, R., Populaire, P., Koenig, F., Myon, J., Pascal, S. and Pasquet, J. (1967): *Arzneimittel-Forsch., 17,* 948.
Kasirsky, G. J. and Tansy, M. F. (1971): *Teratology, 4,* 131.
Kerber, I. J., Warr, O. S. and Richardson, C. (1968): *J. Amer. med. Ass., 203,* 223.
Köhler, E. (1970): In: *Metabolic Pathways in Mammalian Embryos During Organogenesis and its Modification by Drugs,* p. 17. Freie Universität, Berlin.
Krugman, S. and Katz, S. L. (1974): *New Engl. J. Med., 290,* 1375.
Kuenssberg, E. V. and Knox, J. D. E. (1972): *Brit. Med. J., 2,* 292.
Lancet (1974): Editorial, 1, 1489.
Levin, J. N. (1971): *J. Pediat. 79,* 130.
Levy, E. P., Cohen, A. and Fraser, F. C. (1973): *Lancet, 1,* 611.
Lewis, R. B. and Schulman, J. D. (1973): *Lancet, 2,* 1159.
Long, S. Y., (1972): *Teratology, 6,* 75.
Lowe, C. R. (1973): *Lancet, 1,* 9.
McBride, W. G. (1961): *Lancet, 2,* 1358.
McBride, W. G. (1972): *Teratology, 5,* 262 (abstract).
McFarlane, W. V., Pennycuik, P. R. and Thrift, E. (1957): *J. Physiol. (Lond.), 135,* 451.
Meadow, S. R. (1970): *Proc. roy. Soc. Med., 63,* 48.
Mercier-Parot, L. and Tuchmann-Duplessis, H. (1974): *Drugs, 8,* 340.
Milkovich, L. and Van Den Berg, B. J. (1974): *New Engl. J. Med., 291,* 1268.
Miller, R. W. (1969): *Science, 166,* 569, quoting the Atomic Bomb Casualty Commission, 1956.
Nielsen, J., Friedrich, U. and Tsuboi, T. (1969): *Brit. Med. J., 3,* 634.
Noller, K. L., Decker, D. G., Lanier, A. and Kurland, L. T., (1972): *Mayo Clin. Proc., 47,* 629.
Nora, J. J. and Nora, A. H. (1974): *New Engl. J. Med., 291,* 731.
Nora, J. J., Trasler, D. G. and Fraser, F. C. (1965): *Lancet, 2,* 1021.
Nora, J. J., Vargo, T. A., Nora, A. H., Love, K. E. and McNamara, D. G. (1970): *Lancet, 1,* 1290.
Notelovitz, M. (1974): *Lancet, 2,* 902.
Popert, A. J. (1962): *Brit. J. Med., 1,* 967.

Ravid, R. and Toaff, R. (1972): In: *Drugs and Fetal Development*, p. 505. Editors: Klinberg et al. Plenum Press, New York.

Robson, J. M. and Sullivan, F. M. (1963): *Lancet, 1*, 638.

Roux, C. and Dupuis, R. (1961): *C. R. Soc. Biol. (Paris), 155*, 2255.

Roux, C. and Taillemite, J. L. (1969): *C. R. Soc. Biol. (Paris), 163*, 1299.

Rugh, R. (1958): *Pediatrics, 52*, 531.

Rugh, R. (1965): In: *Progress in Radiology*, p. 1356. Editors: L. Turano et al. ICS 105, Excerpta Medica, Amsterdam.

Rugh, R. and Grupp, E. (1960): *Anat. Rec., 138*, 380.

Schaeffer, A. J. (1965): *Diseases of the Newborn.* W. B. Saunders, Philadelphia.

Schou, M., Goldfield, M. D., Weinstein, M. R. and Villeneuve, A. (1973): *Brit. med. J., 2*, 135.

Scott, J. K. (1968): *Lancet, 1*, 208.

Speidel, B. D. and Meadow, S. R. (1972): *Lancet, 2*, 839.

Spira, N., Goujard, J., Huel, G. and Rumeau-Rouquette, C. (1972): *Rev. méd. franç., 41*, 2683.

Stewart, A. (1957): *Proc. roy. Soc. B, 50*, 9.

Sutherland, H. W., Stowers, J. M., Cormack, J. D. and Bewsher, P. D. (1973): *Brit. med. J., 3*, 9.

Tanimura, T. (1972) In: *Symposium on the use of Non-Human Primates for Research in Problems of Human Reproduction*, p. 293. Editors: A. Diczfalusy and C. Stanley. World Health Organization.

Tjio, J. H., Pahnke, W. N. and Kurland, A. A. (1969): *J. Amer. med. Ass., 210*, 849.

Tuchmann-Duplessis, H. (1975): *Concours méd., 97*, 3647.

Tuchmann-Duplessis, H., Hiss, D., Mottot, G. and Rosner, I. (1974): *Thérapie, 29*, 877.

Tuchmann-Duplessis, H. and Mercier-Parot, L. (1962): *Chemotherapia (Basel), 4*, 304.

Tuchmann-Duplessis, H. and Mercier-Parot, L. (1963a): *C. R. Soc. Biol. (Paris), 157*, 1193.

Tuchmann-Duplessis, H. and Mercier-Parot, L. (1963b): *C. R. Acad. Sci. (Paris), 256*, 1841.

Tuchmann-Duplessis, H. and Mercier-Parot, L. (1964a): *C. R. Acad. Sci. (Paris), 258*, 2666.

Tuchmann-Duplessis, H. and Mercier-Parot, L. (1964b): *Bull. Acad. nat. Méd. (Paris), 148*, 392.

Tuchmann-Duplessis, H. and Mercier-Parot, L. (1969): *C. R. Acad. Sci. (Paris), 269*, 2147.

Tuchmann-Duplessis, H. and Mercier-Parot, L. (1972): *J. Gynec. obstet. Biol. Repr. 1*, 141.

Tuchmann-Duplessis, H. and Mercier-Parot, L. (1973): *Nouv. Presse Méd., 2*, 2719.

Wallner, J. J., Waidel, E. and Welsh, H. (1973): *Arch. gynäk., 214*, 83.

Warkany, J. and Takacs, E. (1959): *Amer. J. Path., 35*, 315.

Warrel, D. W. and Taylor, R. (1968): *Lancet, 1*, 117.

Wilkins, L. (1959): *Arch. Anat. micr. Morph. exp., 48 bis*, 313.

Wilson, J. G. (1971): *Fed. Proc., 30*, 104.

Wood, J. W., Keehn, R. J., Kawamoto, S. and Johnson, K. G. (1967): *Amer. J. publ. Hlth., 57*.

Zellweger, H., McDonald, J. S. and Abbo, G. (1967): *Lancet, 2*, 1066.

Congenital disease of late onset

C. O. Carter

Medical Research Council, Clinical Genetics Unit,
Institute of Child Health, London, U.K.

Any genetic defect in an individual will almost invariably have been present from conception, but in general terms there is no difficulty in the concept that a specific defect may not affect development until growth is nearly complete. Only a minority of genes are active in a particular tissue at a particular stage of development. The activity of genes is under the control of other genes and of metabolites in the cytoplasm. It has not yet been shown that control on the Jacob and Monod model applies in mammals, but there is undoubtedly some such control and this is the basis of tissue differentiation. Liver is a tissue with many genes active in producing enzymes; fibrous tissue has a much more limited complement of enzymes.

However, nearly all tissue differentiation is over by the end of the period of post-natal growth and most of it complete at the time of birth. When we look at a genetic disease which has an onset in adult life, we are usually looking at a disease process which, though it has its onset prenatally, only gradually gives rise to sufficient disturbance to cause signs and symptoms.

The types of mechanisms involved may I think be conveniently classified into three groups: (1) genetically determined tissue abnormality which leads to premature failure of function from normal wear and tear with increasing age; (2) sensitivity to particular foods or drugs, such that exposure to these trigger agents is required before signs and symptoms develop; (3) cumulative deposition in tissues of metabolites whose metabolic degradation or removal from the cell is impaired.

In addition, in rather a different category, there are a number of relatively common alleles which do not directly cause disease but which predispose to particular diseases, such that the majority of those who possess the allele never develop the disease and those who do develop the disease often develop it late in life.

Tissue abnormality leading to undue wear and tear

Multiple epiphyseal dysplasia

This condition is autosomal dominant which, in medical genetics, means that patients are heterozygous for the mutant gene involved. As is often the case with dominant conditions, multiple epiphyseal dysplasia shows much variation in age of onset and severity. Pain and stiffness in the knees, elbows, and hips usually develops in childhood. The patients tend to be shorter than unaffected members of the family and to have especially short fingers and toes. The serious disability is the progressive development of osteoarthritis in adult life. In the family shown in Figure 1 (Barrie et al., 1958) all patients were able to work. The grandmother II2 was still ambulant with the help of sticks at the age of 60; III9

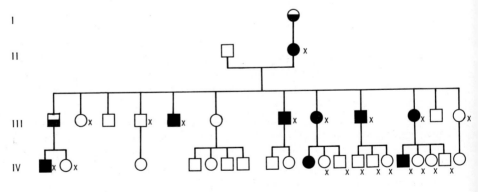

x = x-ray examination

Fig. 1. Pedigree of dominant epiphyseal dysplasia.

only recently had to give up his week-end game of cricket; but IV1 could only walk with difficulty at the age of 20.

The defect in this condition is in the formation and calcification of the epiphyses of the long bones. The epiphyses appear late and radiologically are seen to be small, mottled and to have grossly irregular margins. The basic defect is not known. It is not difficult, however to understand the early development of osteoarthritis in the affected joints with their irregular articular surfaces.

The variation in severity in this and many other dominant conditions is most likely attributable in large part to variation in the corresponding 'normal' gene with which the mutant gene interacts. One tends to think of heterozygotes as having one abnormal mutant gene and one normal gene. But research is showing that at most gene-loci there is 'polymorphism', that is to say that there are several different 'normal' alleles common in the population, as for example, at the ABO blood group locus.

Marfan syndrome

This again is an autosomal dominant condition with marked variation in severity of clinical manifestation. The arachnodactyly, tall stature, scoliosis, joint laxity, ectopia lentis and blue sclerae are present in varying degree in childhood. However the features which endanger life are the lack of resistance of the arterial walls to haemodynamic wear and tear. There develops dilatation of the ascending aorta, incompetence at the mitral valve and dissecting aneurysm of the thoracic or abdominal aorta. These features do not usually develop till the fourth and fifth decade, though aortic regurgitation has been found as early as 10 months and as late as the seventh decade (McKusick, 1972).

Histologically in the wall of the aorta there is sparsity and fragmentation of elastic fibres, whorls of seemingly hypertrophied small muscle, and an increase in collagenous tissue. All these changes are best seen in the ascending aorta, where haemodynamic stress is greatest and where there is the greatest normal physiological dilatation with each ventricular ejection.

The basic defect is not known; it is apparent that there is a connective tissue defect, but not which component of connective tissue is primarily involved. It is a plausible hypothesis that when a mutant gene is dominant, the product of the normal allele at the gene locus involved is a structural protein, as opposed to an enzyme. It will therefore be logical to look at the structure of proteins such as collagen and elastin in this disorder as the appropriate chemical methods become available.

Adult type of polycystic disease of the kidney

This is an autosomal dominant condition in which signs and symptoms usually do not develop until the 4th and 5th decade. The patients present with hypertension and progressive renal failure. Once again there is much variability in manifestation with only very rarely an onset of clinical disease in childhood, while not uncommonly the condition remains asymptomatic throughout life. The malformation is however probably always present from birth.

In a remarkable family in my own experience (Blyth and Ockenden, 1971) the index patient, a girl, presented at the age of 2 years with a severely infected right kidney and was found to have bilateral enlarged kidneys. The infected kidney was removed and found histologically to belong to the dominant adult type of polycystic disease, rather than the autosomal recessive form, which is commoner in childhood. On examination the child's father was found to have mild hypertension and an intravenous pyelogram showed bilateral polycystic kidneys. The mother later had an unplanned pregnancy. At parental request because of the 1 in 2 genetic risk this pregnancy was terminated at 14 weeks. Twin foetuses were found and, on microscopical examination, cortical and medullary cystic tubules were found in all four kidneys.

Sensitivity to food or drugs

Genetic defects which result in sensitivity to food or drugs will be symptomless until the patient is exposed to the exogenous trigger factor.

Glucose-6-phosphate dehydrogenase (G-6-PD) deficiency

The high frequency of the particular mutant gene which is responsible for G-6-PD deficiency in Negroes was not fully appreciated until the introduction of primaquine as an antimalarial drug in the 1950's (Hockwald et al., 1952). The specific enzyme defect was demonstrated a few years later and found to be present in some 14% of Negro males. The gene locus concerned is on the X chromosome. Conditions due to enzyme deficiencies are usually autosomal recessive or X-linked. The relatively rare homozygous women are as much at risk as hemizygous males. It was soon found that these patients were sensitive to other synthetic drugs including some sulphonamides. Naphthalene induces a particularly acute haemolysis.

The Eastern Mediterranean form of G-6-PD deficiency, due to a different gene mutation at the same gene locus, may cause symptoms earlier, because, in addition to sensitivity to a wider range of drugs, patients are sensitive to a common food, the Fava bean. This idiosyncrasy was known to the ancient Greeks. There is remarkable variation in sensitivity between individuals with the defect, which is ill understood, but may depend on other genetic factors.

Porphyria variegata

The South African form of porphyria which Dean and Barnes (1958) have studied so elegantly is autosomal dominant. The incidence in Afrikaaners is about 3 per 1000. Most patients in South Africa may be traced back to a single pair of immigrants from Holland married at the Cape in 1688. This long survival of the mutant gene implies that over the last three centuries it has caused little or no loss of reproductive fitness. Minor symptoms and signs depend on the patient's sensitivity to sunlight; this is usually no more than an inconvenience. However, the introduction of sulphonamides and barbiturates drastically altered the picture. In many of those with the gene these drugs caused attacks of acute abdominal pain and neuropathy which were often fatal.

The basic defect is not precisely known but leads to an increase in hepatic ALA synthetase, perhaps as a consequence of inadequate feed-back repression by heme of the synthesis of this enzyme secondary to loss of intermediary metabolites, such as uroporphyrinogen and coproporphyrinogen, between ALA and heme due to an abnormal cell membrane permeability. These patients continuously excrete protoporphyrin and coproporphyrin in faeces.

Suxamethonium sensitivity

A third example of a genetic condition which is symptom-less until the patient's exposure to a synthetic drug is suxamethonium sensitivity, an autosomal recessive condition. The atypical cholinesterase produced by the more common form of mutant gene is inefficient in hydrolysing suxamethonium, and hence the prolonged and dangerous apnoea when the drug is used as a muscle relaxant.

The accumulation of metabolites

In most autosomal recessive storage conditions, for example von Gierke disease or Tay-Sachs disease, the storage of metabolites in the affected tissues is present at birth, develops rapidly thereafter and leads to death in childhood.

Kinnier-Wilson disease

However, in Kinnier-Wilson disease the accumulation of intracellular copper is slow and about half the patients present in the second and about half in the third decade. The onset of symptoms may range from 6 to 50 years. Canadian workers have suggested that the Eastern European variant has a relatively late onset (Cox et al., 1972). The increased deposition of copper is demonstrable in liver, bone, kidney and cornea. The clinical features may be primarily of liver failure or of dysfunction of the basal ganglia.

The basic defect is not yet precisely known: there is low serum copper, low plasma caeruloplasmin levels, an increased excretion of copper in urine but a decreased excretion in bile, and an increased intestinal absorption of copper. But whatever the basic defect, the accumulation of copper is only slow, perhaps because it is not very closely dependent on the basic, presumably enzymatic, defect.

Fabry's disease

In this X-linked condition there is accumulation of a crystalline glycosphing-olipid, trihexosyl ceramide, in endothelial, perithelial, and smooth muscle cells of blood vessels. Lipid deposits are also prominent in epithelial cells of the cornea and the glomeruli and tubules of the kidney. In the hemizygous male clinical onset is usually in childhood with pain in fingers and toes, telangiectases, corneal opacities and progressive renal failure, but the onset may be only in the second or third decades. In the heterozygous females, however, the disease is much milder and of later onset, though most of them ultimately die of the disease (Burda and Winder, 1967).

The primary defect is a deficiency of ceramide trihexosidase, the enzyme which catabolises trihexosyl ceramide. The slower deposition of trihexosyl ceramide in heterozygous females is to be expected on the Lyon hypothesis, since only a proportion of such females' cells will have as the active X chromosome that with the mutant gene.

Monogenic hypercholesterolaemia

The overall association of hypercholesterolaemia and ischaemic heart disease is well known. The mechanism is not certain but probably involves thrombus formation on patches of arterial atheroma which contain much cholesterol. If hypercholesterolaemia is defined as the upper fifth percentile of the continuous distribution, most cases are multifactorially determined. However, individual families suggestive of monogenic inheritance have long been known. In the patients in these families there is a particularly high risk of early death from ischaemic heart disease. Slack (1969) has estimated that 50% of male patients die by age 60 and that this form is responsible for some 5 to 10% of all such early deaths. The relatively high risk with this monogenic form is very probably due to the fact that, in contrast to the multifactorially determined forms, cholesterol is raised even in childhood. The great majority of patients with this condition are heterozygotes. The rare homozygotes are much more severely affected and usually die of ischaemic heart disease in their late teens or early 20's.

The basic defect has recently been studied in fibroblast culture by Brown and Goldstein (1974). They have demonstrated that fibroblasts from homozygotes lack the capacity to bind low density and very low density lipoproteins. This results in lack of feed-back repression of the synthesis of hydroxymethylglutaryl-CoA reductase, which is the enzyme that controls the rate of cholesterol biosynthesis. Brown and Goldstein suggest that the failure to bind low density lipoproteins in homozygotes is due to a lack of the specific receptor sites on the cell surface. They have found evidence of a partial defect in heterozygotes such that a higher level of plasma lipoprotein is reached before the synthesis of hydroxymethyl-glutaryl-CoA reductase is repressed.

Common alleles predisposing to multifactorially caused disease

The first clear-cut instance of common alleles predisposing to common disease was the association of blood group O, non-secretor, which gives a liability to duodenal ulcer nearly 3 times higher than does group A_1 secretor.

More recently some stronger associations have been found with polymorphic gene loci.

Pulmonary emphysema

Alpha$_1$-antitrypsin, a glycoprotein with a molecular weight of 50,000, is able to enter most body fluids including saliva, lung secretions, duodenal fluid and cerebrospinal fluid. It is active against a wide spectrum of proteolytic enzymes including elastase and a neutral protease of neutrophils. Its functional activity may be measured by antitrypsin activity and its concentration immunologically (Talamo, 1975).

Polymorphism for the gene locus producing the protein is present, with most of the population homozygous for the Pi^m gene (Pi stands for protein inhibitor) and having normal antitrypsin activity. The alleles Pi^s, Pi^z and the rare Pi^- are associated with increasing deficiency of antitrypsin activity. Pi^{zz} homozygotes are about 0.7 in 1000 of the population; their antitrypsin activity is about 20% of normal and about 80% of them will develop emphysema, usually in young adult life, and about 10% will develop infantile hepatic cirrhosis. Pi^{sz} heterozygotes are about 1.4 in 1000 of the population and have about 40% of activity. A smaller but significant proportion will develop emphysema and they will tend to develop it later than Pi^{zz} individuals. Pi^{mz}, about 15 per 1000 of the population, are more likely than the Pi^{mm} individuals to get emphysema; nevertheless most will escape.

Ankylosing spondylitis

90% of patients with ankylosing spondylitis possess the histocompatibility allele HLA B_{27} (formerly called HL-A_{27}), but this is present in only 7% of the population, a relative risk more than 100 times greater in those with the HLA B_{27} allele than in those who do not have it.

Nevertheless, of all males with HLA B_{27} only about 5% get ankylosing spondylitis, and of females with this allele only about 0.5% get the disease. Thus the HLA B_{27} allele is only one of the multifactorial agents causing the disease.

The association might be due to a direct effect of the gene or due to close linkage-disequilibrium with a gene which has a direct effect in causing the disorder. The latter is probably the case since even in affected families (Brewerton, 1975) the linkage is not 100%. The HLA B gene locus is probably very close to the Ia (immune-associated) gene locus, and, as means are found of identifying these, one may expect that the operative association may be with one of the alleles at this Ia locus, but that it is still only part of a polygenic predisposition to develop the disease.

A number of less strong associations with individual alleles at the HLA B locus are being found, mostly with disorders that might be reasonably expected to have an immunological component, such as diabetes, coeliac disease and multiple sclerosis.

In the mouse the Ia genes have been found to control susceptibility to specific virus infections, and it is possible that in diseases such as ankylosing spondylitis and multiple sclerosis it is exposure to a specific virus infection which determines whether those with the specific Ia gene develop the disease.

References

Barrie, H., Carter, C. and Sutcliffe, J. (1958): *Brit. med. J., 2,* 133.

Blyth, H. and Ockenden, B. G. (1971): *J. med. Genet., 8,* 257.

Brewerton, A. D. (Ed.) (1975): *Ann. rheum. Dis., Suppl.*

Brown, M. S. and Goldstein, J. L. (1974): *Proc. nat. Acad. Sci. (Wash.), 71/3,* 788.

Burda, C. D. and Winder, P. R. (1967): *Amer. J. Med., 42,* 293.

Cox, D. W., Fraser, F. C. and Sass-Nortak, A. (1972): *Amer. J. hum. Genet., 24,* 646.

Dean, G. and Barnes, H. D. (1958): *Brit. med. J., 2,* 866.

Hockwald, R. S., Arnold, J., Clayman, D. and Alveng, S. A. (1952): *J. Amer. med. Ass., 149,* 1568.

McKusick, V. (1972): *Heritable Disorders of Connective Tissue,* 4th ed. Mosby, St. Louis.

Slack, J. (1969): *Lancet, 2,* 1380.

Talamo, R. C. (1975): *Paediatrics, 56,* 91.

3: The internal environment of the body

Ultrastructural identification of receptors and binding sites at the cell surface*

L. Orci and A. Perrelet

Institute of Histology and Embryology, School of Medicine, University of Geneva, Switzerland

Receptors and binding sites are functional entities of the cell surface and their localization at the ultrastructural level has become a subject of current interest in cell biology and hormonal research (for review see Kahn, 1975; Oseroff et al., 1973). This brief report will show that three basic techniques of transmission electron microscopy can be used for visualizing receptors or binding sites. All three can be applied to whole cells or to fractions of isolated cell membranes. They are: (1) thin sectioning, which reveals small segments of the cell membrane in cross-section; (2) freeze-fracturing followed by deep-etching (Steere, 1957; Moor et al., 1961; Branton, 1966), which provides an insight into the interior of the cell membrane and a frontal view of small portions of its outer surface; (3) shadow-casting (Smith and Revel, 1972), which yields a frontal view of large areas of the outer surface of the cell membrane. Figures 1 to 4 show examples of images obtained with each of the three preparation techniques.

---

* This work was supported by Grant No. 3.553.75 from the Fonds National Suisse de la Recherche Scientifique, and by a grant-in-aid from Hoechst Pharmaceuticals, Frankfurt.

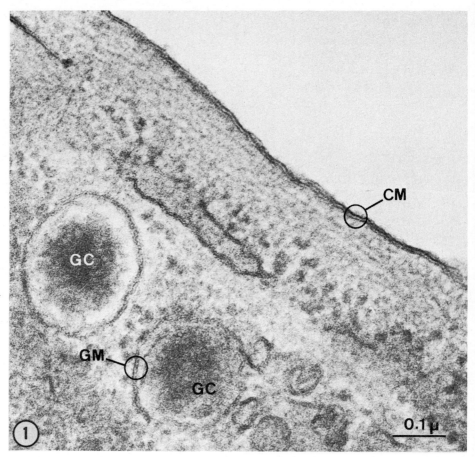

Fig. 1. Periphery of an islet cell in thin section. When the plane of the section is adequate, the plasma or cell membrane (CM) appears as a trilaminar structure consisting of two dense lines and a less dense intermediate layer. A similar structure, the granule's membrane (GM), surrounds the core (GC) of individual secretory granules. × 140,000.

However, since receptors have not so far been shown to have intrinsic contrast or shape that would make them resolvable in their native state by electron microscopy, visualization of them is always indirect and by the use of specific molecules as markers. These can be detected morphologically by their electron density and/or their distinctive shape. Besides the choice of marker, an important step in the visualization process is the coupling of the marker to the mole-

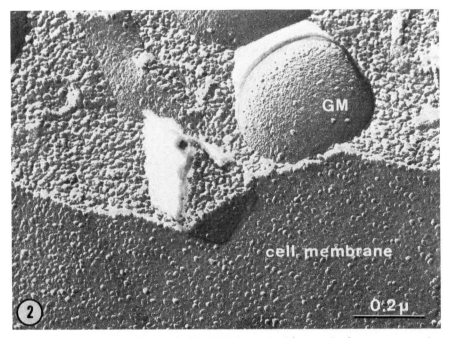

Fig. 2. Periphery of an islet cell in freeze-fracture. In this case the fracture process has exposed the inside of the cell membrane (cytoplasmic leaflet) and shows numerous small protrusions which represent the intramembranous particles (proteins). GM = granule's membrane. × 95,000.

cules (hormones, antibodies, lectins, etc.) specific for the receptor to be demonstrated.

Our two experimental systems are as follows: one is the study of lectin-binding sites in the membranes of pancreatic endocrine cells in monolayer culture; the other consists of localizing the insulin receptors in isolated and purified liver cell membranes. The study of lectin-binding sites in pancreatic monolayer cultures is performed as follows. Concanavallin A (Con A) is added to the culture medium. The cells are then exposed to hemocyanin, a marker molecule for Con A, and prepared for thin sectioning or shadow-casting (Orci et al., 1975a). During the process, Con A first attaches to the lectin-binding sites (which are sugar residues of the cell surface) and is then bound to the hemocyanin molecules. These latter are easily detectable in thin sections or in shadow-cast replicas by their large size (350 Å), shape and electron density (Smith and Revel, 1972).

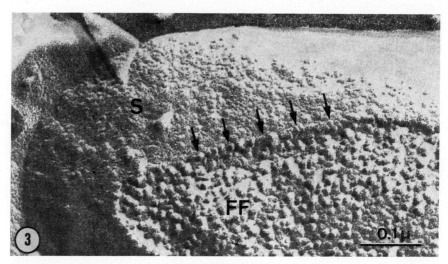

Fig. 3. Isolated cell plasma membrane after freeze-fracture followed by deep-etching. Freeze-fracture has split the membrane (cf. Fig. 2) and exposed its inside with intramembranous particles (fracture face, FF). Subsequent etching has exposed the true surface of the membrane (S), which is devoid of particles. The fracture face and the true surface are separated by a ridge (arrows) representing the thickness of one leaflet of the plasma membrane. × 160,000.

Figure 5 shows a thin section of the periphery of an islet cell of a monolayer culture (Orci et al., 1973) treated sequentially with Con A and hemocyanin at 37°C before glutaraldehyde fixation. While individual hemocyanin molecules (attached to the outer aspect of the cross-sectioned membrane) can be easily visualized, the thin-section image gives no clue as to the repartition of the binding sites in the plane of the cell surface.

Such information is provided in shadow-cast replicas (Figs. 6 and 8a). In such preparations, treated as before at 37°C, the Con A-binding sites revealed by hemocyanin molecules are grouped in patches of variable size separated by areas of marker-free membrane. On the other hand, in cells of monolayer cultures aldehyde-fixed before the addition of Con A and hemocyanin (Figs. 7 and 8c), the binding sites appear randomly distributed on the cell surface. A similar situation is encountered in cells treated with Con A and hemocyanin at 4°C (Fig. 8b). These results are in agreement with those obtained in similar studies (Rosenblith et al., 1973) and suggest that the lectin-binding sites in the native membrane are randomly distributed, while the patching observed at 37°C in unfixed

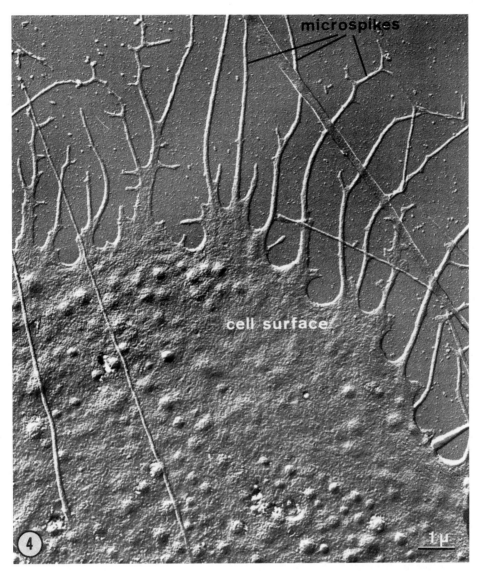

Fig. 4. Periphery of an islet cell in monolayer culture as seen with the shadow-casting technique. This technique reveals the outer surface of the cell membrane; the cell surface has roundish bumps which represent secretory granules bulging from the cytoplasm. The periphery of the cell surface is thrown into several thin processes, the microspikes. ×
10,000.

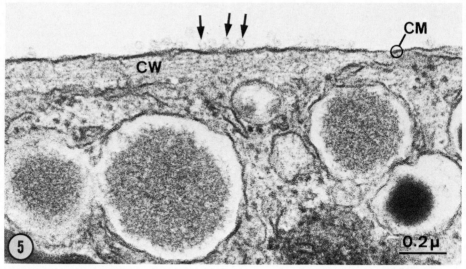

Fig. 5. Thin section of the periphery of an islet cell labeled with Con A and hemocyanin at 37°C before glutaraldehyde fixation. Individual hemocyanin molecules (arrows) reveal Con A-binding sites at the surface of the cell membrane (CM), which is underlined by the microfilamentous cell web (CW). × 65,000.

membrane is induced by Con A*. The specificity of the binding of Con A to glucidic residues of the cell surface is evidenced by the fact that Con A binding can be completely prevented by the addition of α-methyl-glucoside before the application of Con A and hemocyanin (Fig. 9).

The topography of insulin receptors in isolated hepatocyte membranes was studied with ferritin-labeled insulin. The binding to receptors was assessed in thin sections, in freeze-fractured/deep-etched preparations and in shadow-cast replicas (Orci et al., 1975a; Orci, 1975). The ferritin molecule has a diameter of approximately 120 Å, and an electron-dense core of iron. These two properties make it easily detectable in surface replicas and in thin sections. The insulin-ferritin complex was obtained by coupling insulin and ferritin to activated soluble dextran polymers at pH 9 (Bataille et al., 1975). The resulting insulin-

* In view of data obtained in other systems after labeling of surface receptors (Taylor et al., 1971), it is possible that the ligand-induced redistribution of lectin-binding sites in our model is caused not only by a shift of the sites in the plane of the membrane, but also by an internalization of some sites by endocytosis.

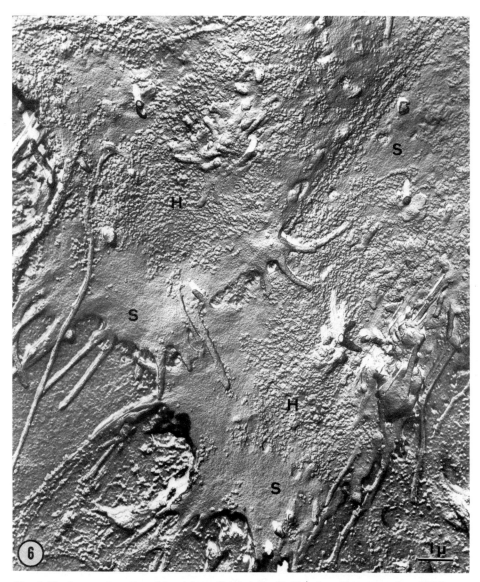

Fig. 6. Shadow-cast replica of two islet cells labeled with Con A and hemocyanin at 37°C before fixation. Patches of hemocyanin molecules (H) are separated by areas of membrane devoid of marker (S). Hemocyanin molecules tend to cover the central part of the cell surface (capping-like distribution). Hemocyanin molecules are noticeably absent from the most peripheral parts of the cells. × 9,000.

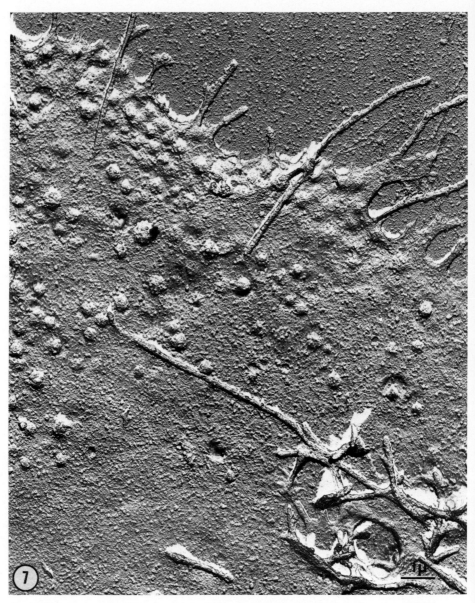

Fig. 7. Shadow-cast replica of an islet cell fixed with glutaraldehyde before the addition of Con A and hemocyanin. In this case, the distribution of the hemocyanin molecules (seen as small protruding dots) is no longer patchy (cf. Fig. 5), but diffuse on the entire cell surface. The roundish bumps represent secretory granules bulging from the cytoplasm. × 9,000.

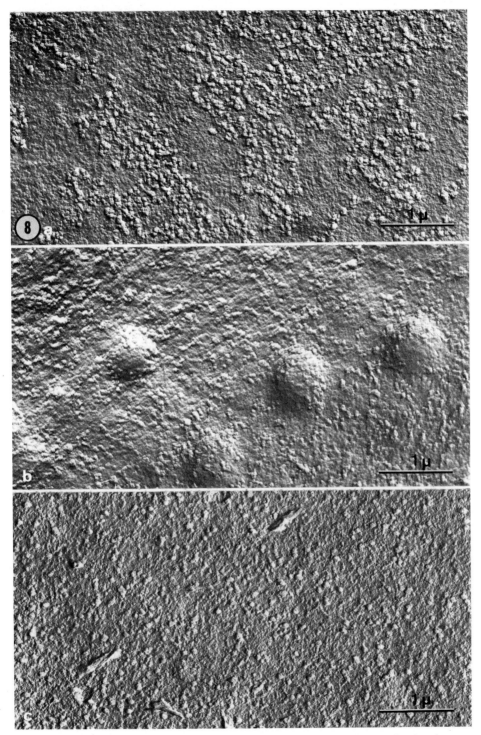

Fig. 8. Portions of islet cell surface in shadow-cast showing at higher magnification the patchy distribution of hemocyanin molecules in cells treated with Con A and hemocyanin at 37°C before fixation (*a*) and the diffuse distribution in cells fixed before Con A-hemocyanin treatment (*c*) (cf. Figs. 6 and 7). The distribution is also diffuse in cells treated with Con A and hemocyanin at 4°C (*b*). × 20,000.

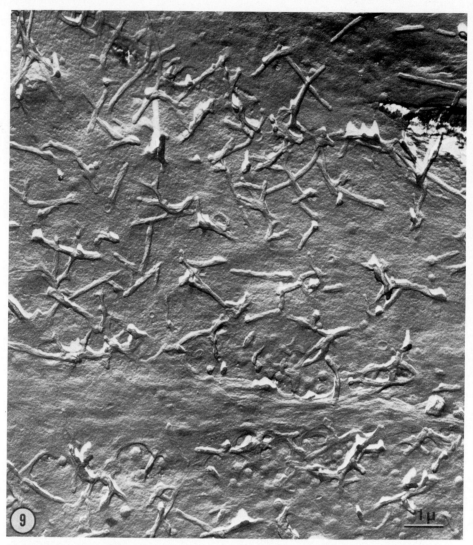

Fig. 9. Shadow-cast replica of an islet cell incubated with α-methyl-glycoside before Con A-hemocyanin treatment. α-methyl-glucoside inhibits Con A-binding, so that practically no hemocyanin molecules are seen on the cell surface. The elongated profiles on the cell surface represent flattened microvilli. × 10,000.

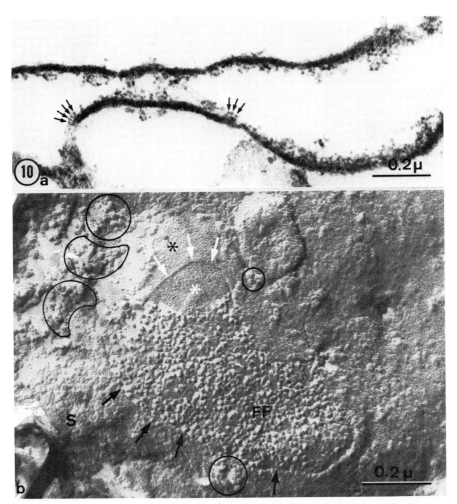

Fig. 10. a: Thin section of isolated liver plasma membrane treated with insulin-dextran-ferritin complex. The dextran-ferritin molecules (arrows) are present in several places on the outer aspect of the plasma membrane. × 80,000. *b*: Freeze-fractured/deep-etched purified liver plasma membrane incubated with insulin-dextran-ferritin complex. Freeze-fracturing has split the membrane and exposed its inside with intramembranous particles (fracture face, FF). Subsequent etching has exposed the outer surface of the membrane (S). The fracture face and the true surface are separated by a ridge (black and white arrows). On the outer surface of the membrane, clusters of dextran-ferritin molecules are outlined in black ink. Note that an area of the fracture face (marked with a white star) is devoid of intramembranous particles and corresponds topographically to a juxtaposed area of the membrane surface (marked with a black star) similarly devoid of dextran-ferritin molecules. (See footnote p. 107) × 95,000.

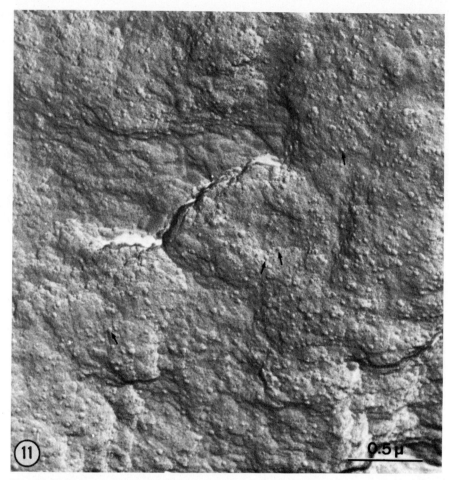

Fig. 11. Shadow-cast replica of purified liver plasma membranes treated with insulin-dextran-ferritin complex. The dextran-ferritin molecules (arrows) are distributed on the membrane surface with a predominantly diffuse pattern. × 40,000.

dextran-ferritin complex, separated from the free insulin by gel filtration, was found to be active in the radioreceptor and radioimmunoassay, and showed the qualitative characteristics of the native hormone. Figure 10 shows the result of labeling liver plasma membranes (isolated according to Neville, 1968) with the insulin-dextran-ferritin complex in thin section (Fig. 10a) and in a freeze-fracture/deep-etch replica (Fig. 10b). Freeze-fracturing splits the membrane

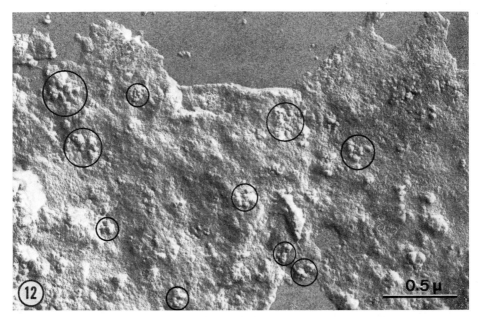

Fig. 12. Shadow-cast replica of purified liver plasma membranes treated with insulin-dextran-ferritin complex. This illustrates the patchy distribution of dextran-ferritin molecules. Clusters are marked by circles. × 40,000.

internally, revealing intramembranous protein particles (Branton, 1971; Vail et al., 1974), while deep-etching exposes the outer surface of the membrane where ferritin molecules can be detected*. In shadow-cast preparations, which allow still larger areas of the membrane to be studied, one sees clearly that labeled zones of the membrane alternate with unlabeled zones. In labeled zones, the binding sites appear either as random, single ferritin-dextran molecules (Fig. 11) or as small clusters of several subunits (Fig. 12). Clusters are separated by a few

* In another study (Orci et al., 1975a; Orci, 1975) we demonstrated clustering of the intramembranous proteins in the fracture face, paralleled by clustering of the insulin-binding sites at the deep-etched outer surface. This was taken as an indication that the insulin receptor, thought to be a glycoprotein (Cuatrecasas, 1971), could be an elongated molecule spanning the entire thickness of the plasma membrane. Such a molecule would thus contribute to the population of intramembranous particles, and have one end (probably the carbohydrate-rich moiety bearing the receptor site) exposed at the cell surface and the other in contact with the cytoplasmic matrix (including the microfilamentous cell web) underlying the inner surface of the cell membrane.

hundred Å and usually contain 3 to 12 molecules. Approximately 12 clusters are present in 1 μm^2. In this respect it is interesting to note that 25 to 60 binding sites per μm^2 of hepatocyte membrane were found in studies in which radioactive insulin was used to measure binding (Orci et al., 1975b). The binding, as revealed in morphological studies, is inhibited by pretreatment of the isolated membrane with free insulin before the application of the insulin-dextran-ferritin complex (Orci et al., 1975a; Orci, 1975).

Further studies are needed to clarify whether this pattern of insulin binding—diffuse and patchy—is inherent in the hepatocyte membrane, or due to the preparative procedure, or the result of reversible clustering caused by the binding of insulin to receptors, as in the case of the ligand-induced redistribution of Con A-binding sites.

Summary

The purpose of this paper is to briefly review two examples of localization of receptor and binding sites at the ultrastructural level. Localization succeeded in thin section, freeze-fracture/deep-etch and shadow-cast preparations; binding sites for lectins were identified with hemocyanin-labeled concanavalin A in monolayer cultures of endocrine pancreatic cells, while receptors for insulin were localized with ferritin-labeled insulin in isolated and purified liver plasma membranes. The results are discussed in the light of relevant literature.

References

Bataille, D., Freychet, P., Rosselin, G. and Orci, L. (1975): Insulin-dextran-ferritin: preparation of an active complex by use of a new protein – protein coupling method. Submitted for publication.
Branton, D. (1966): *Proc. nat. Acad. Sci. (Wash.), 55,* 1048.
Branton, D. (1971): *Phil. Trans. B, 261,* 133.
Cuatrecasas, P. (1971): *J. biol. Chem., 246,* 7265.
Kahn, C. R. (1975): In: *Methods in Membrane Biology, Vol. 3: Plasma Membranes,* p. 81. Academic Press, New York.
Moor, H., Mühlethaler, K., Waldner, H. and Frey-Wyssling, A. (1961): *J. biophys. biochem. Cytol., 10,* 1.
Neville Jr, D. M. (1968): *Biochim. Biophys. Acta (Amst.) 154,* 540.
Orci, L. (1975): In: *Polypeptide Hormones: Cellular Aspects.* Ciba Foundation Symposium No. 41. Excerpta Medica, Amsterdam, in press.
Orci, L., Bataille, D. and Freychet, P. (1975b): *Diabetes, 24, Suppl. 2,* 395.
Orci, L., Like, A. A., Amherdt, M., Blondel, B., Kanazawa, Y., Marliss, E. B., Lambert, A. E., Wollheim, C. B. and Renold, A. E. (1973): *J. ultrastruct. Res., 43,* 270.

Orci, L., Rufener, C., Malaisse-Lagae F., Blondel, B., Amherdt, M., Bataille, D., Frey-chet P. and Perrelet, A. (1975a): *Israel J. med. Sci., 11,* 639.

Oseroff, A. R., Robbins, P. W. and Burger, M. M. (1973): *Ann. Rev. Biochem., 42,* 647.

Rosenblith, J. Z., Ukena, T. E., Yin, H. H., Berlin, R. D. and Karnovsky, M. J. (1973): *Proc. nat. Acad. Sci. (Wash.), 70,* 1625.

Smith, S. B. and Revel, J. P. (1972): *Develop. Biol., 27,* 434.

Steere, R. L. (1957): *J. biophys. biochem. Cytol., 3,* 45.

Taylor, R. B., Duffus, W. P., Raff, M. C. and De Petris, S. (1971): *Nature new Biol., 233,* 225.

Vail, W. J., Papahadjopoulos, D. and Moscarello, M. A. (1974): *Biochim. biophys. Acta (Amst.), 345,* 463.

Control of immune responsiveness: influence of T lymphocytes

J. F. A. P. Miller

Experimental Pathology Unit, The Walter and Eliza Hall Institute of Medical Research, Royal Melbourne Hospital, Melbourne, Australia

In many experimental and clinical situations it would be highly desirable to enhance the immune response or some of its manifestations, e.g. in resistance to some infectious agents and to antigenically distinct tumours. In other situations it would be valuable to suppress the immune response, e.g. in allergic disorders, autoimmune diseases and transplantation of alien skin or organs. A beginning has been made towards the achievement of such goals. For example, the use of adjuvants in immunization is a well established procedure and is a first step towards immunopotentiation. Moreover, the use of specific antibody to suppress the immune response to Rh antigens has been highly successful in the prevention of haemolytic disease of the newborn. Yet effective and safe immunosuppressive agents have still to be found for many clinical conditions and there is also a need for effective and safe adjuvants for use in man. Such deliberate and successful immunomanipulations, in which some arms of the immune response are strengthened and others are weakened, as the circumstances demand, must however await a deeper knowledge and understanding of how the immune system is regulated.

Factors involved in immunoregulation

Immune responses are very complex phenomena and like all physiological processes are subject to homeostatic control. Many factors are involved in regulation of the immune system and result in quantitative as well as qualitative modifications. They may operate at one or several stages of the 'immune reflex arc': (1) they may act on antigen; (2) they may modify the 'afferent arm', i.e. the manner in which antigen is brought to appropriate sites for sensitisation; (3) they may act on the central component – the immunocompetent lymphocytes; and (4) they may modify the 'efferent arm', i.e. the effector function of antigen-activated cells or their progeny. As in all multicellular organisms, factors involved in regulation may be considered at 3 levels: (1) intracellular; (2) intercellular and (3) organismal.

Intracellular regulation operates at the level of the various cells involved in the immune response: T cells, B cells and accessory cells, such as macrophages. Among the factors involved in intracellular regulation are, of course, various gene clusters (McDevitt and Landy, 1972). One type of genetic regulation is mediated by genes which control responsiveness either at the level of antigen recognition or at some step subsequent to this, that is at some step involved in the triggering of a cell that has recognized and bound antigen to its surface. The H-linked Ir genes constitute such a genetic system. Another type of genetic regulation involves genes which control idiotypic determinants, i.e. the fine specificity of the antibody produced. These genes thus presumably code for the variable regions of the immunoglobulin molecule and hence determine the range of specificities for antibody-combining sites. The allotype-linked Ir gene system comprises such genes. Another level of genetic activity determines, not the responsiveness to antigen per se, nor the capacity to elaborate a particular antibody specificity, but the efficiency with which B cells differentiate and proliferate in response to a given antigen. These genes may operate at the level of macrophages and/or B cells. It seems evident that there exist other types of genetic controls. As in other cellular systems, for example, the size of the entire potential progeny of a given antigen-sensitive cell must be limited in some way and this is presumably preprogrammed in the genome.

At the intercellular level, there are large numbers of regulatory factors elaborated and involved in cell to cell interactions (Miller, 1975). The products of one cell influence the behaviour of another cell. This is evident when one considers many of the factors elaborated by the T cell – factors which recruit inflammatory cells by chemotaxis or other means, factors which activate macrophages and enhance their microbicidal activities, and factors which modify B-cell responsiveness by either facilitating or suppressing it (see below). Products of macrophages are also likely to be involved in activating or suppressing T- or B-cell functions. Finally, antibody produced by the B cell itself can act either as an immunopotentiating influence or as a negative feedback turning off the immune response of T cells or of other B cells. There is certainly no single mechanism to account for the phenomenon of immunological tolerance. In fact some forms of tolerance are likely to be the result of one or other modes of immunoregulation. Examples of this are to be found (1) in antibody-mediated tolerance (Diener and Feldmann, 1972), acting at the level of the T cell or the B cell, presumably as a result of antibody complexing with antigen in the right molecular proportions, and (2) in the activities of suppressor T cells which may act on other specific T cells and either directly or indirectly on specific B cells (see below). These and other regulatory mechanisms may be involved in the expulsion or silencing of cells expressing undesirable specificities.

The third level of regulation is organismal. In many multicellular systems, this generally implies regulation by way of the neuro-endocrine system. Much evidence is rapidly accumulating supporting a hormonal control of the lymphoid system (Wolstenholme and Knight, 1970). Humoral influences ('lympho-poietins') are involved at various levels of lymphocyte differentiation from the stem cell to the fully mature T or B cell. Furthermore, growth hormone, steroid hormones, and various other hormones exert effects on the growth and regression of lymphoid tissues. No doubt, humoral mechanisms probably operate to keep the total number of lymphocytes within acceptable limits. For example, surplus cells arising after antigen-induced expansion must be removed to prevent unrestricted growth of lymphocytes, but the discriminating processes involved in such a cellular homeostasis are still far from being understood. Receptors for vasoactive hormones have recently been identified on various subsets of lymphocytes and other leucocytes (Bourne et al., 1974). The β-adrenergic catecholamines, E series of prostaglandins and histamine stimulate the production of cyclic AMP which in turn tends to inhibit the inflammatory or immunological effector function of the cell. Thus, an effect of various hormones via the adenyl cyclase-cyclic AMP system may constitute part of a homeostatic regulation system that limits various immunological effector functions.

The importance of cell interaction in immune responses

The interaction of antigen and immunocompetent lymphocyte is the central feature of an immune response. Generally, however, in order for the reaction to proceed to completion, there is a requirement for a variety of cellular interactions (Table 1). These may occur not only among various classes of lymphocytes

TABLE 1

Cellular interactions in immunity

Collaboration between lymphocytes	T → T T → B	T cells either promote or suppress functions of other T or B lymphocytes
Interaction between lymphocytes and 'accessory' cells	Macrophage ⟨ T B T → macrophage T → polymorphonuclear and mononuclear leucocytes	Antigen presentation Microbicidal activity Recruitment of inflammatory cells

but also between lymphocytes and 'accessory' cells such as mononuclear and polymorphonuclear leucocytes. Collaboration between lymphocytes has now been documented in both cell-mediated and humoral immunity, i.e. between various classes of T lymphocytes as well as between T and B cells. The T cells can either promote or suppress the function of other lymphocytes, depending on the circumstances. Other interactions include macrophage presentation of antigen to either T or B lymphocytes, enhancement of microbicidal activity of macrophages by antigen-activated T cells in cellular resistance to infection, and recruitment of nonspecific mononuclear and polymorphonuclear leucocytes, again by antigen-activated T cells, in cell-mediated reactions such as delayed hypersensitivity. As space does not permit a review of all the various cellular interactions, this presentation will be confined to a discussion of the influence of T cells in controlling B-cell responses.

Requirement for T cells in antibody responses

B cells are antibody-forming cell precursors and antigen-activated B cells will differentiate to antibody-secreting cells (Miller and Mitchell, 1969). It is well known, however, that the antibody response to a variety of antigens is defective in the absence of appropriately stimulated T cells (Miller and Osoba, 1967). Antibody responses highly influenced by T cells are high-affinity antibody production (e.g. secondary responses), IgE and IgG. On the other hand, low-affinity antibody and IgM are marginally or not T-cell dependent (Table 2). There has been a tendency to classify antigens as 'T-dependent' or 'T-independent', and it

TABLE 2

Antibody responses influenced by T cells

Highly T cell-dependent	Marginally or not T cell-dependent
High-affinity antibody IgE IgG	Low-affinity antibody IgM

has been postulated that 'T-independent' antigens can trigger B cells in the absence of T cells because they have a structure which allows them to bind multivalently to the immunoglobulin receptors on the B-cell surface. T-dependent antigens lack such physicochemical characteristics but can bind to antigen recognition sites on T cells. It has been presumed that activated T cells produce and release special immunoglobulin molecules, or IgT, which are cytophilic for macrophages. The macrophage-carrying IgT-antigen complex acts as a matrix to concentrate relevant antigenic determinants in a multivalent manner onto B-cell receptors (Feldmann and Nossal, 1972). According to this hypothesis, therefore, antigen-activated T cells, by secreting specific immunoglobulin molecules cytophilic for macrophages, function essentially as antigen-concentrating devices to encourage effective binding of T-dependent antigens by B lymphocytes. There are several difficulties with such a hypothesis, the major one being the difficulty in unequivocally demonstrating the existence or release of the postulated IgT and its role in collaboration.

Recent work indicates that B cells can indeed be influenced by so-called 'T-dependent' antigens in the absence of T cells. First, antigen binding by B cells is T-cell independent (Ada, 1970). Second, the switch from IgM to IgG expression on the B-cell surface can occur in the absence of appropriately stimulated T cells (Hämmerling et al., 1974). Third, provided the antigen dose is below a certain critical concentration, even memory B cells can be triggered to produce antibody (high affinity and IgG) in the absence of T cells (Klinman and Doughty, 1973). These facts suggest that (a) IgT cannot be an obligatory mediator of collaboration, and (b) the role of T cells in B cell responses is an immunoregulatory one (Mitchell, 1974; Miller, 1975).

Further studies have suggested that B cells with high intrinsic antigen-binding capacity (e.g. IgG rather than IgM producers, or high affinity rather than low affinity) are more susceptible to paralysis (perhaps due to receptor blockade) if antigen tends to persist than B cells with lower antigen-binding potential. This may be the reason why persistent, poorly degradable antigens generally elicit only IgM responses and not IgG. On the other hand, degradable, nonpersistent

TABLE 3

Correlation between antigen persistence, susceptibility to paralysis and absence of T-cell influence*

Antigen persistence	{ carrier:	{ self components, e.g. autologous erythrocytes nondegradable material, e.g. pneumococcal poly-saccharide SIII, poly-D-amino acids
	hapten:	high-affinity hapten-binding capacity of B cells
Absence of T-cell influence	{ athymic mice, T-cell deprived (thymectomized) carrier does not activate T cells	{ self component genetic unresponsive strain chemical peculiarity
Susceptibility of B cells to paralysis	{ high-affinity rather than low-affinity antibody precursor cells IgG rather than IgM precursor cells	

* For further details see Mitchell (1974) and Miller (1975).

antigens elicit both IgM and IgG responses and it is the IgG response and the high-affinity antibody responses which are markedly diminished or abolished in the absence of T cells, the IgM or low-affinity antibody responses being either unaffected or reduced significantly but not abolished. These observations would appear to link (a) antigen persistence, (b) susceptibility of potential IgG or high-affinity antibody producers to paralysis and (c) presence or absence of a T-cell influence (Table 3). By contrast, antigen concentration hypotheses, such as the IgT-macrophage proposal referred to above, infer that B cells with lower antigen-binding potential would have their capacity to bind antigen increased by activated T cells or their products. This implies that, under such circumstances, low-affinity antibody production would be enhanced. This, however, is not the case, so that one is forced to abandon such proposals.

There is much evidence to suggest that the influence by which T cells modify B-cell responsiveness to antigen is nonspecific with respect to the antigenic determinants which activate T and B cells in the system used. The evidence for a nonspecific influence of activated T cells modifying B-cell responsiveness in vivo has been obtained in systems in which a large number of T cells were activated to an irrelevant antigen, as, for example, by injecting allogeneic lymphocytes, the so-called 'allogeneic effect' (Katz, 1972).

In summary, it may be said that any B cell can bind antigen via its immunoglobulin determinants in the absence of any T-cell influence. However, B cells with high antigen-binding capacity (i.e. those B cells that have the potential to produce high-affinity antibody in particular, or IgG antibody in general) are readily paralyzed in the absence of T cells. Conversely, B cells with lower antigen-binding capacity (such as cells producing low-affinity antibody in particular and IgM antibody in general) are not as easily paralyzed by antigen in the presence or in the absence of T cells, possibly because antigen can readily dissociate from their receptors. T cells are activated by antigen generally only if such antigen is presented on some surface such as the cell membrane of a macrophage. Antigen bound to immunoglobulin determinants on B cells seems to be very effective in activating T cells. It may thus be assumed that under normal in vivo conditions, antigen bound to immunoglobulin determinants on B cells recruits T lymphocytes reactive to other determinants of the antigen. Possibly the T cells recognize the B cells bearing antigen-immunoglobulin complexes as foreign cells and are activated to produce nonspecific factors just as in cellular immunity. Among such factors are some which influence the mobility of phagocytic cells and the degradation of antigens by phagocytes. This must lead to removal of antigen from the microenvironment of the B cells and hence protect high-affinity cells from paralysis. Other factors are presumably enzymes, such as proteases, which can activate components of the complement system. Such components have been implicated in triggering of B cells either by acting as an obligatory signal for cell transformation (Dukor and Hartmann, 1973) or by effecting release of antigen-antibody complexes bound to the B-cell membrane (Miller et al., 1973). It is proposed, therefore, that T cells modulate B-cell responsiveness mainly by means of nonspecific factors, which are active only at short distances, and which therefore exert their effect only if the relevant T and B cells are in close proximity, as they would be if antigen molecules linked their receptors.

T-cell suppression of B-cell responsiveness

The possibility of a suppressor effect of T cells on B-cell responsiveness became evident when it was found that cells from tolerant animals could be mixed with cells from normal animals and prevent these from producing antibody to the specific antigen (Gershon, 1974). Further evidence for the existence, in tolerant animals, of T cells which exert an active suppressor effect on IgG antibody production has been obtained by our group (Basten et al., 1974, 1975). Specific immunological tolerance was induced in CBA mice with a single injection of deaggregated chicken or human gammaglobulin. The unresponsive state was stable on adoptive transfer and not reversed after pretreatment of tolerant cells with trypsin. Tolerant cells could suppress the IgG response of normal spleen cells or primed B cells in an adoptive transfer system although the sup-

TABLE 4

Possible mechanisms of T cell-dependent suppression

T cell-dependent antibody:	{ IgG feedback { Antigen-antibody complexes (blocking factors)
'Suppressor' T cells:	{ Anti-idiotypic or anti-allotypic { 'IgT'-antigen complexes blocking B cells { Suppressive substances: specific or nonspecific { Excess helper activity

pression was dose-dependent, low doses facilitating the response, higher doses suppressing it. Incubation of the tolerant cell population with an antiserum that kills T lymphocytes reversed the suppressor effect.

Some of the possible mechanisms of T cell-dependent suppression are listed in Table 4. On the basis of present evidence, it cannot be stated with certainty whether or not suppressor and helper T cells are distinct categories of T cells. Thus, either of the following is possible:

1. Two classes of T cells exist, one facilitating immune responses, the other suppressing them. The recent claim for an enhanced antibody response following passage of normal or primed spleen cells through columns of histamine-rabbit serum albumin-coated sepharose supports the idea that suppressor T cells may be a distinct class of T cells (Shearer et al., 1972).

2. Only one class of T cells exists and suppressor activity results from excessive production of T-cell factors – the 'supra-priming hypothesis'. If this hypothesis is correct, one may predict that high doses of primed T cells might suppress rather than facilitate B-cell responses and that primed T cells would reinforce the suppressor effect of tolerant T cells. On the other hand, should primed T cells abrogate the suppressor effect of tolerant T cells, the possible existence of two distinct types of T cells, one with facilitating and the other with suppressor activities, will have to be seriously considered.

Further clarification is required concerning the target of suppressor activity. In delayed hypersensitivity, it appears that T cells themselves can suppress other T cells (Zembala and Asherson, 1973). In antibody formation, it is not known whether the suppressive effect is exerted directly on B cells, via macrophages, or on other T cells which would have facilitated the response of B cells. There is one case in which B cells producing a particular allotype have been shown to be the targets for suppressor T cells (Herzenberg et al., 1973). This may, however, represent a special situation.

Conclusions

Experiments performed in the last 15 years have certainly increased our knowledge of the physiology of the thymus and its relation to the rest of the lymphoid system. The thymus is responsible for the construction of a pool of recirculating long-lived immunologically competent small lymphocytes or T cells. The discovery of the immunological function of the thymus in 1961 has led to a better understanding of immunological deficiency diseases which afflict man. These can now be classified according to whether the T-cell system, the B-cell system or both are deficient. Replacement therapy, for instance implantation of thymus tissue, has been used with some success in some of these cases (Peterson et al., 1965). Measures which selectively deplete the T-cell population, for instance antilymphocyte serum, impair the capacity to reject foreign tissues –a function of the T cell. Such agents have already been used in our clinics to prevent rejection of organ grafts such as kidney transplants.

By virtue of its capacity to recirculate, the T cell is particularly well equipped for the task of seeking antigen and influencing the response of other lymphocytes and accessory cells. Support for such a role derives from the recent demonstration of rapid and complete recruitment of specific antigen-sensitive cells from the recirculating pool into regions where antigen has been deposited (Sprent et al., 1971; Sprent and Miller, 1974). This occurs during both cellular immunity and humoral immunity. The ensuing interactions within lymphoid tissues between antigen-activated T lymphocytes and effector cells – monocytes, macrophages, granulocytes or B lymphocytes – result in amplification of the immune response. This is manifest by simultaneous triggering of a wide range of host defence systems, constitutive as well as adaptive, including phagocytosis, microbicidal activity, the inflammatory response, kinin release and complement and coagulation cascades.

The T cell-B cell collaboration is the best characterized of the cellular interactions. There is compelling evidence for a crucial role of T cells in determining the amount, class and affinity of the antibody produced by B cells. Indeed the switch from IgM to IgG production and the rise in affinity of the antibody produced both seem to be under T-cell control.

The knowledge that T lymphocytes regulate the activities of other lymphocytes and leucocytes has great significance and practical implications in manipulation of the immune response:

1. Methods are available to augment the activities of T lymphocytes. These include presentation of antigen in the appropriate form or by the appropriate route, and the use of adjuvants such as the Calmette-Guerin bacillus, or of the allogeneic effect. Such procedures, aimed at augmenting T-cell function, should

enhance cellular immunity, microbicidal activity of macrophages and antibody production by B cells. They may thus be beneficial in anergic states characterized by deficient T-cell functions, in various infectious diseases such as leprosy, and in augmenting the efficacy of vaccinating procedures.

2. The suppressive effect of T cells on B-cell responsiveness and on other T-cell activities must be considered in the pathogenesis of autoimmune diseases. Further understanding of the mechanism of action of suppressor T cells might conceivably lead to the control of some of these disorders.

3. The antibody response of B lymphocytes (particularly IgG and IgE) can be turned off by antigenic determinants conjugated to materials (which can be synthesized) that are nondegradable, long-persisting and not T-cell activating. This should provide a new approach to combat allergic disorders or complications (e.g. to penicillin) and possibly autoimmune diseases.

4. In some forms of cancer, where tumour cells have a distinct individual antigenicity of their own, the production of blocking factors may conceivably be diminished if the particular B cells secreting enhancing antibody could be turned off by using one of the above methods.

A major unknown in all these systems is of course the identity of the various antigenic determinants concerned. Clearly, therefore, further detailed studies are required, not only in order to unravel precisely the many factors which activate or suppress T- or B-cell functions, but also to determine the chemical constitution of allergens, tumour-specific antigens and other relevant cellular components. Such a knowledge may eventually allow precise immunological engineering and its application to clinical medicine.

References

Ada, G. L. (1970): *Transplant. Rev., 5,* 105.

Basten, A., Miller, J. F. A. P. and Johnson, P. (1975): *Transplant. Rev., 26,* 130.

Basten, A., Miller, J. F. A. P., Sprent, J. and Cheers, C. (1974): *J. exp. Med., 140,* 199.

Bourne, H. R., Lichtenstein, L. M., Melmon, K. L., Henney, C. S., Weinstein, Y. and Shearer, G. M. (1974): *Science, 184,* 19.

Diener, E. and Feldmann, M. (1972): *Transplant. Rev., 8,* 76.

Dukor, P. and Hartmann, K. U. (1973): *Cell. Immunol., 7,* 349.

Feldmann, M. and Nossal, G. J. V. (1972): *Transplant. Rev., 13,* 3.

Gershon, R. K. (1974): *Contemp. Top. Immunobiol., 3,* 1.

Hämmerling, G., Masuda, T. and McDevitt, H. O. (1974): *J. exp. Med., 137,* 1180.

Herzenberg, L. A., Chan, E. L., Ravitch, M. M., Riblet, R. J. and Herzenberg, L. A. (1973): *J. exp. Med., 137,* 1311.

Katz, D. H. (1972): *Transplant. Rev., 12,* 141.

Klinman, N. R. and Doughty, R. A. (1973): *J. exp. Med., 138,* 473.

McDevitt, H. O. and Landy, M. (Eds.) (1972): *Genetic Control of Immune Responsiveness.* Academic Press, New York.

Miller, G. W., Saluk, P. H. and Nussenzweig, V. (1973): *J. exp. Med., 138,* 495.

Miller, J. F. A. P. (1975): *Ann. N. Y. Acad. Sci., 249,* 9.

Miller, J. F. A. P. and Mitchell, G. F. (1969): *Transplant. Rev., 1,* 3.

Miller, J. F. A. P. and Osoba, D. (1967): *Physiol. Rev., 47,* 437.

Mitchell, G. F. (1974): In: *Progress in Immunology II, Vol. 3,* p. 89. Editors: L. Brent and J. Holborow, North-Holland Publishing Co., Amsterdam.

Peterson, R. D. A., Cooper, M. D. and Good, R. A. (1965): *Amer. J. Med., 38,* 579.

Shearer, G. M., Melmon, K. L., Weinstein, Y. and Sela, M. (1972): *J. exp. Med., 136,* 1302.

Sprent, J. and Miller, J. F. A. P. (1974): *J. exp. Med., 139,* 1.

Sprent, J., Miller, J. F. A. P. and Mitchell, G. F. (1971): *Cell Immunol., 2,* 171.

Wolstenholme, G. E. W. and Knight, J. (Eds.) (1970): *Hormones and the Immune Response.* Ciba Foundation Study Group No. 36. Churchill, London.

Zembala, M. and Asherson, G. L. (1973): *Nature (Lond.) 244,* 227.

4: The external environment of the body

Clinical aspects of the effects of ionizing radiation

Toshiyuki Kumatori

Division of Radiation Health, National Institute of Radiological Sciences, Chiba-shi, Japan

The recognition of the effects of radiation on man began with the discovery of X-rays in 1895. Within a year of the discovery of X-rays various ill effects, which included conjunctivitis, erythema, swelling and necrosis of the skin, alopecia, and chronic skin lesions, were reported. In 1897 attention was directed to the acute symptoms. In 1902 a case of cancer was recorded following chronic ulceration caused by X-rays. Many data concerning radiation effects on man have been accumulated, supported by animal experiments, but our knowledge is still insufficient. The comprehensive reports of the United Nations Scientific Committee on the Effects of Atomic Radiation have been published (1958, 1962, 1964, 1966, 1969, 1972).

Exposure

Radiation exposure is classified into two types, external and internal. External exposure arises from a source emitting radiations capable of travelling some distance through the air. In this case X-rays, gamma-rays and neutrons are important. Internal exposure is much more complicated. The radiation source must be in a form capable of entering the body. Radioactive substances enter through inhalation, ingestion or a wound in the skin. In this case alpha-emitters and beta-rays play a large role in the grade and type of radiation effects. There are cases in which external and internal exposure coexist.

Sources of information on human exposure

We have at present few sources of data on human exposure. The main ones are as follows: (1) occupationally exposed groups; (2) medical diagnostic and therapeutic exposure; (3) a limited number of people in various types of radiation accidents; (4) atomic bomb survivors in Japan; (5) a group exposed to fallout radiation in 1954.

Besides the investigations on these groups many experiments have been done to increase our knowledge of the effects of ionizing radiation.

Effects

Radiation effects are called 'somatic' if they become manifest in an exposed individual, and 'genetic' or 'inherited' if they affect his descendants.

Usually radiation effects are classified into 'acute' and 'late'. While acute effects occur soon after the initial exposure, late effects appear after a latent period which can extend up to many years.

The causal relationship between acute effects and radiation is relatively clear. However, in the case of late effects, that relationship is usually obscure. One of the reasons is that most diseases due to late effects of irradiation are usually indistinguishable from diseases normally arising in a population or those due to other causes, i.e. there are no 'radiation-specific' changes. Another reason is the long latent period after the initial exposure.

The evidence in man that radiation may be the cause of events occurring long after exposure is based on their significantly increased incidence in the exposed group as compared to an adequate unexposed control group.

Factors that influence the effects

Radiation effects can be influenced by several factors. The Joint Report of the Industrial Medical Association Radiation Committee and the Workmen's Compensation Committee (1960) described these as follows:

1. The effects of external radiation will vary mainly depending upon (a) the

absorbed dose; (b) the dose rate; (c) the distribution of the dose in time (continuous over a period or intermittent) and space (within organs and tissues); (d) the extent of exposure – whole body or partial; (e) the sensitivity to radiation of the tissue or system exposed; (f) the biological effectiveness of the radiation for the tissue considered; (g) the type and energy of the radiation; and (h) the nature of the effect being considered.

2. The effect of a radioisotope deposited in the body will vary depending upon: (a) the site of deposition in the organs; (b) the half-life of its radiation and the time of retention in the organ; (c) the type and energy of the radiation emitted; (d) the sensitivity of the critical organ or tissue to radiation injury; and (e) the essentiality of the organs affected.

Acute effects

These effects include the relatively prompt biological changes arising from large doses and can range from barely detectable to grossly deleterious changes. At above 100 rads and up to a median lethal dose (300 to 500 rads) hematological changes are prominent. Above this dose and up to about 2,000 rads gastrointestinal damage is predominant. At extremely high exposures, i.e. several thousand rads, the central nervous system is damaged. At 600 or more rads mortality will be high.

Local acute effects include skin damage and temporary or permanent sterility. These effects will probably lead to chronic damage.

Chromosome abnormalities

Recent developments in methods for detecting changes in the frequency of chromosome aberrations have made it possible to estimate the absorbed dose biologically to as low as 10 rads. Figure 1 shows the evolution of the chromosome aberration rate and estimated dose in a case accidentally exposed to ^{192}Ir gamma-rays (Ishihara et al., 1973). On the basis of the yields of dicentrics and rings, estimates of the average absorbed dose were made by using the dose-response relations for ^{60}Co gamma-rays and for Linac X-rays (Sasaki, 1971). The dose was equivalent to 124 rads of ^{60}Co and 152 rads of Linac X-rays. The technique for more close estimates of the effects of uneven exposure was applied in the same case. The frequency of dicentrics in X_1Cu cells (cells with unstable chromosome abnormalities which are in their first cell division since exposure) and their Qdr value should be extrapolated on the dose-response relationships of high-energy X-rays in vitro in the estimation (Sasaki and Miyata, 1968; Sasaki, 1971). The Qdr values at various times after exposure were almost

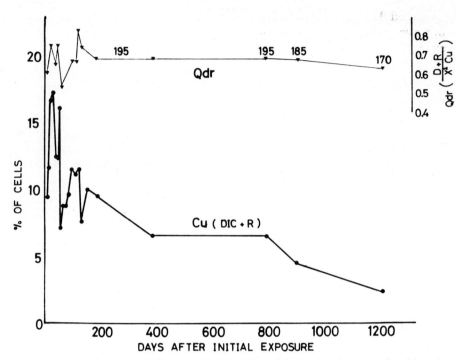

Fig. 1. Shifts with time in the frequency of Cu cells and Qdr values in a case of accidental exposure to [192]Ir. The numbers above the Qdr line indicate the averaged total body doses absorbed (rads) obtained from the Qdr values.

constant, and the estimated doses were higher than those obtained by direct extrapolation from the aberration yields. The chromosome aberrations are very sensitive, and even many years after it is possible to make a crude estimate of the absorbed dose from their frequencies.

The other main clinical and pathological observations on the acute effects are summarized below in the section on the Bikini radiation accident, with the results of follow-up studies over a 20-year period.

Late effects

Statistical methods are useful in determining the degree of probability of a causal relationship between exposure to radiation and late effects such as the development of leukemia and other malignancies etc. As a result of investigations into the incidence in exposed human groups, the following diseases or

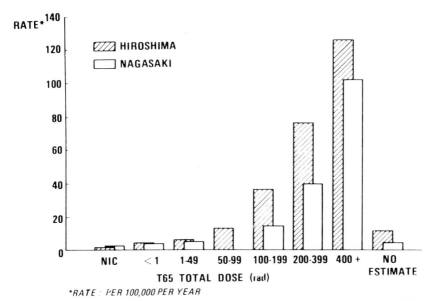

RATE*

*RATE : PER 100,000 PER YEAR

Fig. 2. Incidence of leukemia in atomic bomb survivors. (From Ichimaru and Ishimaru, 1975; courtesy of the editors *J. radiat. Res.*).

conditions are now considered the main late effects: leukemia, thyroid cancer or nodule, breast cancer, lung cancer and fibrosis, bone necrosis and neoplasia, skin cancer, liver cancer or cirrhosis, cataract and sterility. Besides these, mental and growth retardation and microcephaly have been observed among atomic bomb survivors. Animal experiments have also shown the life-shortening effect.

The incidence of leukemia in atomic bomb survivors in Hiroshima and Nagasaki is shown in Figure 2 (Ichimaru and Ishimaru, 1975). This is the crude annual incidence of leukemia (all types) between October, 1950 and December, 1971 by city and dose categories. There seems to be a linear relationship between the incidence and doses over 100 rads in Nagasaki and 50 rads in Hiroshima. However, below these levels nothing is known for sure. There is no evidence that the risk of leukemia has returned to control levels in the survivors who received a significant dose. In relation to leukemogenic effects of radiation, one has to take into account the quality of radiation, the subject's age at the time of exposure and the time elapsed since exposure.

Genetic effects in man have not been proved. However, irradiation of the germ cells may cause mutations which manifest themselves in later generations.

Including genetic effects, no conclusive answer is available to the question whether there is a threshold dose of radiation below which damage does not occur. At present it seems prudent to assume, for the purposes of radiation protection, that there is no threshold and that a linear relationship exists between dose and effects, even with the smallest dose.

Findings in the Japanese fishermen exposed to fallout in 1954

On March 1, 1954, 23 Japanese fishermen aged between 18 and 39 were exposed to radioactive fallout produced by the thermonuclear test explosion performed by the U.S. authorities at Bikini lagoon. At the same time 239 Marshallese and 28 Americans were exposed to the fallout produced by the same test explosion.

The location of the boat was 166° 58′ E. and 11° 53′ N. At about 3.50 a.m. they saw a huge red light in the west. They heard detonation-like sounds 7-8 minutes later while they were fishing for tuna. At about 7.00 a.m. white ashes began to fall on the boat and this continued for about $4\frac{1}{2}$ hours.

After 14 days' they returned to their harbor, Yaizu, on March 14. After landing, all the fishermen were found to have been injured by the radioactive material. They were hospitalized by March 28, and were discharged from hospital in May 1955, except one fatal case who died on September 23, 1954. After being discharged, most of them have been examined so far as possible on an annual basis. Several surveys have since been reported (Miyoshi and Kumatori, 1955; Koyama et al., 1955; Mikamo et al. 1956; Kumatori and Miyoshi, 1963; Kumatori et al., 1964; Kumatori, 1971; Ishihara and Kumatori, 1967, 1969).

State of irradiation and estimated radiation dose

When the fallout was most intense they could not keep their mouths and eyes open. The fallout deposit on the deck was so thick that their foot prints showed in it. They were irradiated in the following ways: (1) from radioactive materials adhering to the skin; (2) externally from the radioactive materials in the cabins and on the deck, etc.; (3) internally from the radioactive materials that entered various organs.

The specific activity of the fallout at 7.00 a.m. on March 1 was estimated as 1.4 Ci/g. The estimation of the radiation dose to the skin and by internal exposure was difficult. On the other hand, the estimated external radiation dose was approximately 170-600 rads for 14 days, about half or more being irradiated on the first day (Table 1). The dose received by each person differed according to his behavior on the boat and the position of his cabin.

TABLE 1

Estimated dose (rads) of whole body gamma radiation

Subject No.	1st day	Total	
T- 1	240-290	450-500	
T- 2	210-260	390-440	
T- 3	150-200	260-310*	(310-410)
T- 5	400-430	660-690	
T- 6	130-180	200-250	
T- 7	140-190	220-270	
T- 8	310-360	520-570	
K- 1	190-220	310-340	
K- 2	130-180	200-250	
K- 3	140-190	230-280	
K- 4	120-170	190-240	
K- 5	140-190	220-270	
K- 6	180-230	300-350	
K- 7	230-280	340-390	
K- 8	220-270	380-430	
K- 9	310-360	550-600	
K-10	140-190	230-280	
K-11	120-170	170-220	
K-12	100-150	170-220	
K-13	250-300	370-420	
K-14	420-500	510-590	
K-15	140-190	210-260	
K-16	120-170	190-240	

* T-3 put the fall-out material close to his bed.
Therefore, about 100 rads should be added in total.

The integrated dose to the thyroid glands from ^{131}I was inferred as about 20-120 rads. Urine samples collected 4 weeks after the explosion revealed a significant amount of radioactivity. However, the radioactivity decreased rapidly and by about 6 months after the explosion it was barely detectable. In the analyses made after $8\frac{1}{2}$ years and 10 years the urinary levels of ^{137}Cs and ^{90}Sr were the same as in normal Japanese. At that time the results of whole-body counting showed no significant difference between these fishermen and controls. The radioactivity in several organs of the fatal case was low but still higher than in controls.

Clinical and laboratory findings

General symptoms and signs
Soon after the initial exposure most of the fishermen experienced anorexia, fatigue and lachrymation, and in some cases nausea and vomiting occurred.

Skin lesions
Skin lesions were caused by beta irradiation. Shortly after the exposure, they suffered from erythema followed by edema, vesiculation, erosions, ulceration or necrosis. Epilation was observed in 20 cases, especially in 2 who did not wear hats while the ash fell and lost all their hair. These skin lesions were histologically similar to ordinary radiodermatitis. The skin injuries healed gradually. Now, 20 years after the exposure, a few cases still show depigmentation, pigmentation and capillary dilatation. Atrophy of the epidermis with narrowing of the stratum granulosum were clearly seen in histological sections of these areas examined 10 years after the exposure.

Hematology
Leukocytes: The total number of leukocytes decreased gradually, showing the lowest count at 4-8 weeks. In 5 cases the count was less than 2,000/mm^3; in 13 it was less than 3,000 and in 5 it was less than 4,000. In one case, the leukocyte count fell to 800. A correlation was found between the minimum neutrophil

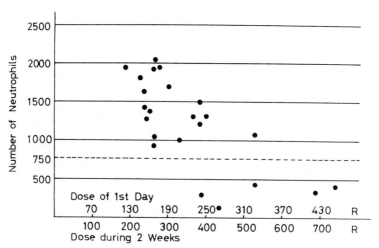

Fig. 3. Correlation between minimum neutrophil count and dose of gamma radiation.

count and the externally irradiated gamma dosage (Fig. 3). Initial lymphopenia was followed by marked neutropenia. After 8 weeks recovery was clear, though many cases showed remarkable eosinophilia at that time. In some cases slightly immature neutrophils appeared in the peripheral blood.

Erythrocytes: Severe cases showed slight anemia accompanied by reticulocyte depression. The color indices were over 1.0. The Price-Jones curves were at first displaced to the right of normal, but returned to almost normal after one year.

Platelets: Platelet counts showed an increasing depression, reaching a minimum at 4-7 weeks (15,000-100,000/mm^3). Slight coagulation disturbances were observed in a few cases.

Bone marrow: In severe cases the bone marrow was highly hypoplastic at the critical stage, but changed to slightly hypoplastic and then almost normoplastic. Recovery was not complete even after a year. The coexistence of hypoplastic and hyperplastic areas was observed in histological sections at the recovery stage. These changes were seen even in examinations made 10-15 years after the exposure.

Morphological abnormalities: Several morphological abnormalities, e.g. abnormal granules in the lymphocytes or neutrophils, vacuoles in various leukocytes and megakaryocytes, giant nuclei and hypersegmentation of neutrophils, binuclear lymphocytes, abnormal mitosis of erythroblasts etc., were observed

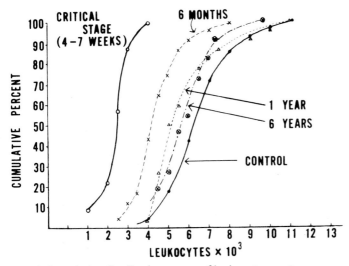

Fig. 4. Cumulative distribution curves of leukocyte counts.

for about one year, especially at the critical and recovery stages. A small increase in 'mitotically connected abnormalities' was found in the bone marrow smears of a few cases after 10 years.

Recovery: The cumulative distribution curves of the leukocyte, erythrocyte and platelet counts were displaced to the left of normal ones, particularly at the critical stage. Though the erythrocyte and platelet curves lay on the normal Japanese ones after 2 years, the leukocyte curve was still displaced slightly to the left of normal after 6 years (Fig. 4).

Cytogenetics

Follow-up of chromosome observations in blood cells has been performed since 1964. Even 20 years after exposure, cells with chromosome abnormalities (both Cu and Cs cells) were much commoner in the peripheral lymphocytes than in the general population. The frequency of Cu cells (dicentrics and rings), however, was decreasing. On the other hand, Cs cells remained fairly constant at a frequency of around 2% (Table 2). The frequency of chromosome abnormalities was found to correspond with the severity of the injuries, as indicated by the minimum neutrophil count at the critical stage. In the bone marrow, cells with chromosome abnormalities (Cs cells) were found quite constantly at frequencies greater than 2% in all 4 samplings carried out 13-17 years after exposure. In some cases clone formations were proved.

The estimates of the absorbed dose based on chromosome abnormalities showed a crude correlation with the physical estimates.

TABLE 2

Incidence of chromosome abnormalities in peripheral lymphocytes of the Bikini fishermen (data from 1966, 1967, 1969 and 1974)

Sample (no. of patients)	No. of cells examined	% Cu cells	% Cs cells
1966 (10)	750	0.67	1.20
1967 (13)	950	0.74	2.11
1969 (14)	4138	0.41	1.86
1974 (12)	12000	0.19	
	2373		2.15
Control 1	9510	0.02	0.07
2	608	0.00	0.16

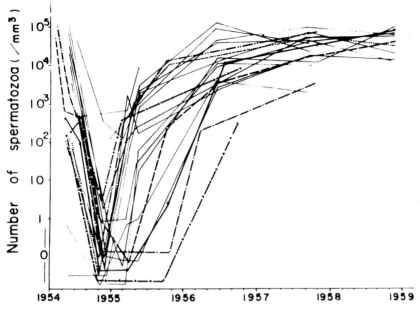

Fig. 5. Changes in the number of spermatozoa over 5 years.

Spermatopoiesis

The number of spermatozoa decreased about 2 months after exposure. Reduced motility and morphological abnormalities were also observed in the spermatozoa. Indications of recovery were seen about 2 years after exposure (Fig. 5), and most of the patients had healthy children.

The testicles of the subject who died 206 days after exposure showed extremely reduced spermatopoiesis.

Other findings

Slight disturbances of liver function were found in a few cases at the time of hospitalization. Later these became more obvious. One of the fishermen, who showed remarkable hematological disturbances, died from liver damage. During follow-up studies elevated GOT and GPT values were observed in several cases. In 1974, ascites was proved in 2 cases. In one of them (T-7) this was accompanied by diabetes mellitus and sepsis. While T-7 has now recovered, the other case (K-6) died from liver cirrhosis in April, 1975. It is difficult to prove the existence of a relationship between the exposure and the liver damage.

Ophthalmological examinations showed slight lenticular opacities in several cases. The significance of this is not yet apparent. Other studies, including thyroid studies, are continuing to detect late effects.

Excellent reports have been published on the exposed Marshallese. One of the remarkable late effects is the appearance of thyroid nodules in the survivors who were exposed at under 10 years of age. About 76% of these people had thyroid nodules. One of them died of acute leukemia in 1972 (Conard et al., 1970; Conard, personal communication, 1974).

Conclusion

Since the peaceful uses of atomic energy are being developed, research on the effects of low-level radiation has been required recently. However, we lack information about its effects in man. Both experimental studies and observations in man are necessary to get information for extrapolation from present knowledge, obtained from animal experiments and surveys of men exposed to high-dose radiation, to low-level effects. At the same time adequate measures for radiation accidents are needed because accidents can be expected in many new circumstances.

References

Conard, R. A. et al. (1970): BNL 50220 (T-562), Brookhaven National Laboratory, Upton, New York.
Ichimaru, M. and Ishimaru, T. (1975): *J. Radiat. Res., 16, Suppl.,* in press.
Ishihara, T. and Kumatori, K. (1967): In: *Human Radiation Cytogenetics,* p. 145. Editors: H. J. Evans, W. M. Court Brown and A. S. McLean. North-Holland Publishing Co., Amsterdam.
Ishihara, T., Kohno, S., Hirashima, K., Kumatori, T., Sugiyama, H. and Kurisu, A. (1973): *J. Radiat. Res., 14,* 328.
Ishihara, T. and Kumatori, T. (1969): *Jap. J. Genet., 44, Suppl. 1,* 242.
Joint Report of the Industrial Medical Association Radiation Committee and Workmen's Compensation Committee (1960): *J. occup. Med., 2,* 503.
Koyama, Y., Kumatori, T. et al. (1955): *Iryo, 9,* 1.
Kumatori, T., Ishihara, T., Ueda, T. and Miyoshi, K. (1964): *Medical Survey of Japanese Exposed to Fallout Radiation in 1954.* National Institute of Radiological Sciences, Chiba.
Kumatori, T. and Miyoshi, K. (1963): In: *Diagnosis and Treatment of Radioactive Poisoning,* p. 253. International Atomic Energy Agency, Vienna.
Kumatori, T. (1971): In: *Biological Aspects of Radiation Protection,* p. 64. Editors: T. Sugahara and O. Hug. Igaku Shoin, Tokyo.
Mikamo, Y. et al. (1956): In: *Research in the Effects and Influences of the Nuclear Bomb*

Test Explosions, Vol. II, p. 1313. Japan Society for the Promotion of Science, Tokyo.

Miyoshi, K. and Kumatori, T. (1955): *Acta haemat. Jap., 18,* 379.

Sasaki, M. S. (1971): In: *Biological Aspects of Radiation Protection,* p. 81. Editors: T. Sugahara and O. Hug. Igaku Shoin, Tokyo.

Sasaki, M. S. and Miyata, H. (1968): *Nature (Lond.), 220,* 1189.

United Nations Scientific Committee on the Effects of Atomic Radiation: Report. General Assembly Official Records, XIII Session, Suppl. 17 (A/3838) (1958); XVII Session, Suppl. 16 (A/5216) (1962); XIX Session, Suppl. 14 (A/5814) (1964); XXI Session, Suppl. 14 (A/6314) (1966); XXIV Session, Suppl. 13 (A/7613) (1969); XXVII Session, Suppl. 25 (A/8725) Ionizing Radiation: Vol. 1: Levels; Vol. II: Effects (1972).

Environmental exposure and cancer

John R. Goldsmith*

*Epidemiological Studies Laboratory,
California State Health Department, Berkeley, Calif., U.S.A.*

One of the most feared consequences of the introduction of new physical and chemical agents is that after a decade or so evidence will be found that the introduction led to a new cause of cancer. The fear is increased by the concern that such carcinogenicity will persist and impair the lives and comfort of many innocent and healthy persons.

The prediction of environmental cancer hazard is a task engaging experimental pathologists, among others. The task of monitoring for the occurrence and trend in cancer by site and cell type among exposed populations is one for the anatomical and surgical pathologist, cooperating with cancer registries. Clinical pathologists help to estimate proximate effects of exposure. Early detection by cytological methods is a contribution of the cytologists. The faint hope that methods for reducing the risk of cancer in those who have been exposed is nurtured by the work of experimental oncologists.

This opportunity to review with you an epidemiologist's view on environmen-

* Based on work initiated during assignment to the Office of the Associate Director for Field Studies and Statistics, National Cancer Institute, Bethesda, Md.

tal causes of cancer is thus welcome, for it is the interaction of epidemiologist and pathologist which has brought us to our present appreciation of environmental cancer and which will offer the best hope of managing the real problems and abating the fear engendered by the reality of environmental causes of cancer.

To illustrate this we may note that an unambiguous diagnosis of adenocarcinoma of the maxillary sinus, angiosarcoma of the liver, mesothelioma of the pleura and peritoneum, melanoma of skin, oat cell cancer of the lung, or clear cell carcinoma of the vagina can be reached by one or more pathologists. But the knowledge of the excessive frequency of such cases in persons exposed to, respectively, hardwood furniture-making, vinyl chloride, asbestos in the work place or home, sunlight, bis-chloromethyl ether, or stilbestrol therapy of the mother in pregnancy is provided by epidemiologists. Both together become concerned with validity, completeness of ascertainment, and timeliness of notification and prevention. Yet most of these are examples of rare cancers and we still must concern ourselves with the more common and preventable associations, among which occupational exposure to cancer-causing agents ranks high.

I propose to discuss the ways in which our knowledge about agents, occupations and types has accumulated; then I shall consider what proportion of human cancer is environmentally caused and the prospects for improving detection and prevention using established methods or new approaches which will enable us to offer hope instead of anxiety to those who have been at risk.

Geographical pathology

Geographical differences in cancer incidence have been used as clues to environmental effects for about 25 years, since the 1950 U.I.C.C. meeting in Oxford. A series of reports from the U.S. National Cancer Institute on cancer mortality for 1950-1969 by county for the U.S. is a suitable way to commemorate the anniversary. Sir Richard Doll's work and analyses dominate this period. In his Rock Carling Fellowship volume, Doll (1967) pointed out that for men aged 35-64 in areas of the world with reasonably comparable cancer registration or certification, geographical differences of 50 to 1,000 times occur for cancer of the liver, esophagus, penis, nasopharynx, and lip. Cancer of trachea, bronchus and lung is not far behind, with a gradient of 40 between the highest incidence areas, Liverpool and Birmingham, and Uganda and Ibadan, Nigeria, the lowest areas. Such gradients imply environmental gradients, possibly interacting with genetic factors. Kuratsune et al. (1974), observing high rates of lung cancer in one area of Japan, were able to identify a high risk ratio for employees in an arsenic-producing metal smelter. Previous observers in the community had not drawn the conclusion that smelter work increased the risk of lung cancer. Blot and Fraumeni (1975), basing their data on the 20-year county cancer mortality study, showed that both men and women had higher lung cancer rates in communities with copper, lead or zinc smelters. They attribute this to exposure to arsenic.

Geographical pathology is also a hypothesis-generating form of analysis. For example, from the county mortality data maps have been derived for 35 anatomic sites. For two sites, trachea-bronchus and lung, and for lymphosarcoma a tendency for a coastal excess among men but not women is observed (Mason et al., 1975). For trachea-bronchus and lung the excess occurs along the South Atlantic and Gulf coasts, and certain industrial areas. For lymphosarcoma, the excess is along the coast of California and Connecticut and New York excluding the areas where lung cancer is high. The occupational basis is suggested because the female rates do not show such an excess. Among the highest counties for white male lymphosarcoma is Clatsop county, Oregon, but for mapping in order to have a sufficiently large population at risk, its data for lymphosarcoma were merged with adjacent counties with a much greater population, including the city of Portland, and the resulting area has a rate which is average. This illustrates the problem of dilution, which may make geographic pathology fail to show, in the combined experience of a large population, an excess among a small subpopulation.

Alert, clinical observation as a detection method for environmental cancer

Most of the known occupational risks and chemical carcinogens were first identified by alert clinicians, who observed a small number of cases, usually of a rare form or site of cancer, among a population with a common occupation or exposure. This was the case with bladder cancer excess among dyestuff workers, clear cell cancer among women whose mothers had stilbestrol during pregnancy, angiosarcoma of the liver among men exposed to work in vinyl chloride polymerization, and adenocarcinoma of the sinus among hardwood furniture workers, to name a few. Here the pathologist may be able to play a critical role if an unusual cell type begins to appear in his case registry. By calling the clinicians or occupational health authorities to ask if there may not be a common occupational experience or environmental exposure behind this cluster, an individual pathologist can discover a new carcinogenic hazard. The 'alert practitioner', to borrow a phrase from Dr. Robert Miller, Chief of Epidemiology of the National Cancer Institute, is the key to improved detection of environmental cancer (Miller, 1969).

Cancer registries and industrial cohort studies

A network of local, national and international cancer registries is evolving which serves many purposes, including estimation of incidence, evaluation of treatment or prognosis and, to an increasing degree, the detection of occupational or environmental cancer hazards. On an international level, the International Agency for Research on Cancer in Lyon and the International Association of Cancer Registries provide a coordinating mechanism and in September 1975, in cooperation with the National Cancer Institute, held a workshop and training course on Cancer Registries and Occupational Cancer.

For example, the collection of occupational exposure histories among persons having reports of bladder or head and neck cancer can be proposed, coordinated and coded by cancer registries. One group in Los Angeles has established a system of identifying relatively uncommon cancer types, sites, or ages for extensive follow-back history of exposure using cancer registry staff and by permission of the referring physician. Another method, for which pioneering work was done by Dunn et al. (1960) in California, is to match occupationally defined groups with the reported cancer experience collected by a population-based registry. This initial work, using mortality data alone, identified increased risk of lung cancer in sheet metal workers exposed to asbestos and in restaurant cooks.

An independent, but similar development has been the follow-up of occupational groups for which a hazard has been suspected in order to see to what extent specific jobs and exposures and preventive methods are influencing cancer experience. This type of procedure is often based on labor union or union-management agreements.

Examples include the cohort studies of asbestos insulation workers in the U.S. which have identified the potent interaction of cigarette smoking and asbestos exposure in lung cancer, the excess of gastrointestinal cancer and of laryngeal cancer and the high rates of mesothelioma among persons exposed to asbestos (Selikoff et al., 1973).

Lloyd (1971) and his colleagues have demonstrated by this type of procedure the excess lung cancer rates among coke-oven workers. Using Norwegian cancer registry data, Pederson (1973) has shown excess lung cancer among nickel smelter workers and Landgard and Norseth (1975) have shown excesses among zinc chromate pigment workers. Spitzer et al. (1975) have shown that high rates of lip cancer in Newfoundland are due to exposure in fishermen, but specific agents or practices have not yet been identified. Currently, in the U.S. a cooperative union-management-university programme is following a large population of workers in the rubber industry and has shown, among other risks, an association between leukemia rates and exposure to solvents. For example, in one plant lymphatic leukemia occurred in eight men aged between 40 and 64 when about one would be expected. McMichael et al. (1975), by matching cases with high, medium and low exposure to solvents based on detailed job-description exposure records, showed that high exposure to solvents in the 1940-1960 period carried a ninefold excess risk. For the tire-repair job title, there was a sixfold excess risk. Swabbing of tires with solvent was thought to produce the exposure, and the solvent predominantly used in the past was benzene (benzol).

Epidemiological analysis of vital statistical data

The final method of detecting occupational and environmental cancer is through the analysis of vital statistical data. In a sense this interacts with or underlies other methods, especially geographical pathology.

A most extraordinarily valuable analysis of occupational mortality by social class and occupation is made every ten years by the British Office of Population Censuses and Surveys. For married women, analysis is based on the husband's occupation. Table 1 shows occupations with a significantly high 't' test for men and for both men and wives. In the latter category, social class or non-occupational factors are likely to play a role.

In 1963 the U.S. Department of Health, Education and Welfare published an occupational mortality study based on 1950 census data. It needs to be repeated. A comparison of three large scale occupational cancer studies, two from the U.S. and one from the U.K., showed substantial agreement on occupation site associations (Guidotti and Goldsmith, in preparation). The results are shown in Table 2.

Migrant studies

Studies among migrants have been especially useful in yielding clues as to cultural or dietary factors in cancer. The most notable series is that of Haenzsel and Kurihara (1968), which shows the drop in gastric cancer among Japanese populations migrating to Hawaii and to California. This is regrettably associated with a rise in colorectal and breast cancer. In the U.S., Mancuso and Coulter (1958) studied cancer rates among migrants from other countries and found that migrants usually have rates intermediate between those in the populations in the home country and the U.S. Of great interest is their finding of high rates of lung cancer among the black population migrating to the northern industrial state of

TABLE 1

Sites of fatal cancer distinguishing occupations with high 't' values for men and for both men and wives (England and Wales, 1961)*

Site	High in men	High in men and wives
Malignant neoplasm of:		
Lung, bronchus and trachea	Glass and ceramics makers Furnace, forge, foundry, rolling mill workers Electrical and electronic workers Construction workers Painters and decorators Warehousemen, storekeepers, packers, bottlers	Engineering and allied trades workers Food, drink and tobacco workers Transport and communications workers
Kidney	Electrical and electronic workers	
Bladder and other urinary organs	Gas, coke and chemical workers Transport and communications workers Warehousemen, storekeepers, packers, bottlers	
Melanoma of skin	Electrical and electronic workers Food, drink and tobacco workers	
Bone (including jaw bone)	Furnace, forge, foundry, rolling mill workers	
Lymphosarcoma and reticulosarcoma	Clothing workers	
Mouth	Textile workers	
Esophagus	Food, drink and tobacco workers Transport and communications workers	
Stomach	Gas, coke and chemical workers Furnace, forge, foundry, rolling mill workers Painters and decorators Warehousemen, storekeepers, packers, bottlers	Miners and quarrymen Engineering and allied trades workers Textile workers Drivers of stationary engines, cranes Transport and communications workers
Large intestine except rectum	Professional, technical workers, artists	
Rectum	Furnace, forge, foundry, rolling mill workers Textile workers	
Pancreas	Clothing workers	
Peritoneum and unspecified digestive organs	Administrators and managers	
Larynx	Food, drink and tobacco workers	

* Source: Office of Population Censuses and Surveys (1971).

TABLE 2

Extent of agreement between three major studies on occupational cancer excess for selected sites and occupations*

	Mine operatives	Glass and ceramic operatives	Farmers and farm laborers	Chemical production operatives	Chemical production workers	Shoemakers	Leather production workers	Boilermakers	Machinists	Sheet metal workers	Construction painters	Non-construction painters	Textile spinners & weavers	Textile laborers	Cabinetmakers	Carpenters	Woodworkers	Sawyers	Lumbermen
Cancer all sites	Axx	xbx	xxx	xbx	ABx	ABx	aBx	ABc	ABC	ABC	ABC	xBx	axx	ABx	xxc	xxC	xxx	xxx	aox
Cancer of respiratory tract	Axx	aBx	xxx	abc	xBo	ABx	abx	ABc	AxC	ABc	ABC	obc	xxx	ABx	xBx	aBC	oox	xxx	oox
Cancer of digestive tract	Aox	aox	Aoc	aox	xoo	aoC	aoc	aox	AoC	aoC	Aoc	aox	AoC	xox	aoo	AoC	xoo	xox	oox
Stomach cancer	ABo	axo	Axo	oBo	obo	abc	xbo	abo	Axo	Abo	ABo	aoo	abo	oBo	axo	axo	ooo	axo	ooo
Cancer of genito-urinary system	aox	oox	xox	ooc	ooo	ooo	oox	ooc	Aoc	ooo	aoc	ooc	ooo	oox	oox	xoC	ooo	oox	ooc
Buccopharyngeal cancer	aoo	oox	xox	ooo	ooo	ooo	ooc	ooo	Aoo	ooC	aoc	Aoo	ooo	ooo	ooo	xox	ooo	ooo	ooo
Leukemia	Aoc	ooc	xoC	ooc	ooo	ooo	ooc	ooo	aox	oox	aox	ooo	ooc	ooc	ooo	xoC	ooo	ooc	ooo
Lymphoma	Aox	oox	xoc	ooo	ooo	ooo	oox	ooc	Aox	oox	aoc	Aoo	ooo	ooc	ooc	xoC	ooo	oox	oox

Capital A, B and C = significant excess cancer. Lower case a, b and c = non-significant excess cancer (significance defined as P < 0.05). x = not increased, o = not available or insufficient data.

* U.S. Department of Health, Education and Welfare (1963, 1967), Office of Population Censuses and Surveys (1971).

Ohio; Haenzsel et al. (1962) showed earlier that, allowing for cigarette smoking, migrants to urban areas in the U.S. had higher lung cancer rates than life-long residents. This is one piece of evidence against the urban excess of lung cancer being due to community air pollution. Recent work by Menck et al. (1974) and by Henderson et al. (1975) shows high rates of lung cancer in portions of Los Angeles county which are heavily industrialized. This may be due to occupational exposure or pollutants in the community. The former is more likely since the excess is only among men.

The agents involved in environmentally caused cancer

While agents, occupations and industrial exposure give the most direct clues to cancer risks, the biological reality is that interactions of genetic susceptibility and multiple agents are necessary to produce cancer.

One of the best known determinants is skin pigmentation, which seems to protect against skin cancer. Fears et al. (1976) have recently pointed out how much the incidence of melanoma increases with decreasing latitude. This reflects the effects of sunlight exposure on light-skinned populations. The apparent high susceptibility of Japanese to gastric cancer and of some Chinese populations to nasopharyngeal cancer appear from migration data to have a cultural basis. Bjelke's (1973) work on Norwegian migrants is consistent with nutritional deficiency as a basis for high gastric cancer rates in Scandinavian populations.

The most devastating of carcinogenic exposures is that due to cigarette smoking, and for many of the occupational hazards it also has a more than additive interaction with occupational exposure – this is well documented for asbestos and lung cancer and for radon exposure in uranium mines and lung cancer. Since bladder cancer is also increased in cigarette smokers, smoking may have an interactive role with the occupational agents causing bladder cancer, principally organic amines.

From a review of evidence on known human environmental carcinogens, it is clear that nearly all have been identified because of excessive frequency of occurrence of cancer in environmentally exposed human populations.

Table 3, from the International Agency for Research On Cancer (Tomatis, 1975), lists seventeen chemicals and classes of chemicals for which exposure can be causally related to cancer in man. Of these only stilbestrol was first shown to be carcinogenic in animals prior to its carcinogenic effect on women being documented. The carcinogenicity of vinyl chloride and bis-chloromethyl ether was known, but the fact was not published prior to the first human cases being recognized. For arsenic compounds, animal carcinogenicity has yet to be proven, although human carcinogenicity is well documented.

TABLE 3

Chemicals linked to cancer in humans (International Agency for Research on Cancer)

Chemical	Type of exposure	Target organ(s)	Route of exposure
Aflatoxin*	Dietary	Liver	Oral
4-Aminobiphenyl	Occupational	Bladder	Inhalation, oral
Arsenic compounds	Occupational medicinal	Skin, lung	Oral, inhalation
Asbestos (Crocidolite, Amosite, Chrysotile)	Occupational	Lung and pleural cavity, gastro-intestinal tract	Inhalation, oral
Auramine (aurothioglucose)	Occupational	Bladder	Oral, inhalation, skin
Benzene	Occupational	Bone Marrow	Inhalation, skin
Benzidine	Occupational	Bladder	Inhalation, oral, skin
Bis (chloromethyl) ether	Occupational	Lung	Inhalation
Cadmium oxide	Occupational	Prostate	Inhalation, oral
Chromium (chromate-producing industries)	Occupational	Lung	Inhalation
Hematite (Mining)	Occupational	Lung	Inhalation
2-Naphthylamine	Occupational	Bladder	Inhalation, oral
Nickel (nickel refining)	Occupational	Nasal cavity, lung	Inhalation
N,N'-Bis (2-Chloroethyl)2-naphthylamine	Medicinal	Bladder	Oral
Soot and tars	Occupational	Lung	Inhalation
	Environmental	Skin (scrotum)	Skin contact
Stilbestrol	Medicinal	Vagina, uterus	Oral
Vinyl chloride	Occupational	Liver, brain, lung	Inhalation, skin

* Strongly suspected, but not proved.

Additionally, ionizing radiation is known to be carcinogenic, with sunlight, radon daughters and X-rays being the major types of exposures; skin, bone marrow and lung are the commonest target organs.

This list is constantly being added to and clarified, through the work of experimental pathologists and of epidemiologists, and the list of suspected carcinogenic agents, those for which there is some suggestive experimental evidence, is at least ten times as great. The most comprehensive source of information on these agents is a series of monographs being published by the International Agency for Research on Cancer (Lyon, France) entitled 'Evaluation of Carcinogenic Risk of Chemicals to Man, Vols. 1-9', which has so far given an authoritative evaluation for 192 substances.

The proportion of cancer with environmental causes

When we put the question, 'What proportion of human cancer is environmentally caused?', the data are even more difficult to interpret. Answers range up to 80%, based on projections from locations at which cancer rates for each site are unusually low. We must by our studies attempt to see to what extent the gradients can be explained by environmental factors such as sunlight, occupation, diet or community pollution. When considering occupational and other environmental causes, smoking and drinking practices must be allowed for, as cigarette smoking has a substantial impact on frequencies of lung and bladder cancer, and drinking of distilled spirits is associated with increased frequency of esophageal cancer. Hoover and Fraumeni (1975) recently examined the association of cancer mortality in US counties with the presence and type of chemical industry. They found that bladder cancer showed strong positive gradients associated with counties in which there was manufacturing of dyes, dye intermediates and organic pigments, pharmaceutical preparations, perfumes, cosmetics, and other toiletries.

For lung cancer, positive gradients were associated with the manufacture of industrial gases, pharmaceutical preparations, soaps and detergents, paints, inorganic pigments, and synthetic rubber. Liver cancer rates were associated with counties in which synthetic rubber, soaps and detergents, cosmetics and other toiletries and printing ink were manufactured. The authors note that one county (Hamilton, Ohio) accounts for a number of the associations. Elevated lung cancer rates among both men and women are observed in counties with non-ferrous metal smelters, suggesting that smelter emissions have a carcinogenic effect on women with no occupational exposure. Chemical industry counties in such studies may have 10 to 40% excess cancer, which compares with the three- to several hundred-fold excess observed for populations exposed to some of the chemicals in Table 3. Geographic gradients, as shown by the demonstration by Kuratsune et al. (1974) of high rates in metal smelter workers in Japan, can uncover specific occupations at high risk.

However, geographical gradients in cancer mortality along with occupational cancer mortality (U.S. Department of Health, Education and Welfare, 1963; Office of Population Censuses and Surveys; Milham, 1975) provide leads. The environmental scientist, experimental pathologist, and epidemiologist must follow these leads until a specific preventable exposure is identifiable. At present we have more leads than detectives and so many environmental cancer culprits remain at large.

At present, based on 'sound etiological hypotheses', the proportion of cancer at selected sites due to exogenous factors is as shown in Table 4 (Higginson and Muir, 1974).

TABLE 4

Proportion (%) of cancers at selected sites for which there are sound etiologic hypotheses

Site (ISC. 7th revision in parentheses)	Exogenous factors				Congenital familiar or acquired	Un-known
	Cul-tural	Occupa-tional	Iatro-genic	Misc-ellaneous		
Mouth (140, 141, 143, 144)	90	1	—	5	—	<5
Salivary gland (142)	—	—	—	—	—	100
Esophagus (150)	80	—	—	4	<1	±15
Stomach (151)	4	—	—	1	—	95
Colon and rectum (153, 154)	—	—	—	1	<1	99
Liver (155.0)	70	—	—	1	—	30
(155.0) Africa	—	—	—	—	—	100
Lung (162)	80	1-2	—	±8	—	<10
Breast (170)	—	—	—	—	—	100
Cervix uteri (171)	—	—	—	—	—	100
Corpus uteri (172)	—	—	—	—	—	100
Ovary (175)	—	—	—	—	—	100
Other female genitals (176)	—	—	<1	—	—	99
Prostate and testis (177, 178)	—	—	—	—	—	100
Penis (179.0)	—	<1	—	95	—	<5
Bladder (181.0) W. Industrial	50	10-20	<1	—	—	30-40
(181.0) Africa	—	—	—	50	—	50
Skin (190, 191)	—	2	—	80	10	<8
Brain tumors (193)	—	—	2	—	<1	98
Leukemia and lymphoma (200-205)						
Children	—	—	<7	—	1	92
Adults	—	—	<1	—	—	99

Higginson and Muir (1974).

Possible areas for future work based on present knowledge

What, then, are the major obstacles to identification and control of exposure to environmental carcinogens? The long latent period (10 to 30 years) and long lifespan of man compared to experimental animals is one. The relative resistance of humans to cancer due to environmental agents is another. The multiplicity and non-specificity of agents is a third.

Ambiguity as to magnitude and type of exposure is a fourth. The last obstacle I shall list has a favorable aspect; this is the complexity of what is known of the carcinogenic process.

The favorable aspect is that many human carcinogens have non-malignant reactions, which, if properly interpreted, can provide a basis for preventing their malignant effects. Radon exposure in underground mines and bis-chloromethyl ether exposure in the chemical industries produce marked increases in bronchitis symptoms; presumably reducing exposure enough to prevent these bronchitic reactions will go far to prevent malignancies due to these agents. Many of the occupations with high lung cancer rates also have high rates of bronchitis, asthma or emphysema (Table 5) (U.S. Department of Health, Education and Welfare, 1963).

Since many known carcinogens can be shown to be mutagens, there is great interest now in developing rapid tests for mutagenicity, in the hope that avoidance of exposures producing mutagenic reactions will be a useful guide to avoiding exposures which are carcinogenic. Animal tests for carcinogenicity, if they are adequately done, may take a year or two, and cost many thousands of dollars. Tests for bacterial mutagenicity take a few days, and are relatively inexpensive.

TABLE 5

Numbers of deaths and standardized mortality ratios (SMR) for selected occupational groups exhibiting excess mortality from malignant and non-malignant respiratory disease, Males, 20-64, U.S. 1950

Occupational group	Mortality from malignant neo-plasm trachea, bronchus and lung		Non-malignant respiratory disease other than influenza and pneumonia	
	Deaths	SMR	Deaths	SMR
Barbers, etc.	95	151**	29	126
Cooks, except private household	91	165**	41	195**
Machinists and job setters	190	138**	66	125
Molders, Metal	34	227**	30	500**
Painters (construction), paperhangers and glaziers	212	167**	64	133**
Taxicab drivers and Chauffeurs	77	188**	36	225**
Laborers, wood products, etc.	414	138*	20	154
Laborers, primary metal industries	82	167**	49	258**
Laborers, transportation equipment	30	200**	26	433**
Operatives, etc. primary metal industries	77	145**	41	195**

* SMR significantly above 100 at $P \leqslant 0.05$.

** SMR significantly above 100 at $P \leqslant 0.01$.

First priority for future work should, therefore, be given to better definition and validation of laboratory tests for early warnings of the hazard of human carcinogenicity.

A second area for emphasis is the use of cancer registries to pinpoint the types of cancer occurrence which suggest a contribution by environmental exposures, and following them up with occupational and exposure history and measurement. The National Cancer Institute, in cooperation with pathologists in many countries, has assisted in the development of population-based and hospital cancer registries. The use of such systems for obtaining and using data on environment and cancer can provide a much needed basis for monitoring the occurrence and guiding the prevention of environmental cancer.

Thirdly, of great interest but of uncertain value is the finding by experimental oncologists that, if animals are exposed to potent chemical carcinogens, the manifestation of cancer may be prevented if another chemical agent is administered. The class of agents which has received the greatest attention is the retinoids, especially cis-retinoic acid. These agents appear to play a role in regulating epithelial cell differentiation (Maugh, 1974). While side effects of certain members of the class are known, it is believed that they spontaneously disappear when use of the agent is terminated. Should such agents prove to be useful in preventing the manifestations of cancer in human populations at high risk due to environmental exposures, then a stunning advance in cancer prevention will have been made. The possibility of interventive trials with this class of agents is under cautious consideration – awaiting further toxicity evaluation and protocols for the joint goals of protecting the subjects from harm and discerning as early as possible what value can be found from the use of such agents.

References

Bjelke, E. (1973): *Epidemiologic Studies of Cancer of the Stomach, Colon, and Rectum with Special Emphasis on the Role of the Diet, Vol. I.* Doctoral Dissertation, University of Minnesota, School of Public Health.

Blot, W. J. and Fraumeni Jr, J. F. (1975): *Lancet, 1,* 142.

Doll, Richard (1967): *Prevention of Cancer – Pointers from Epidemiology.* Rock Carling Fellowship, Nuffield Hospital Trust, London.

Dunn Jr., J. E., Linden, G. and Breslow, L. (1960): *Amer. J. Publ. Hlth, 50,* 1475.

Fears, T. R., Scotto, J. and Schneiderman, M. A. (1976): *Amer. J. publ. Hlth,* in press.

Haenzsel, W., Loveland, D. B. and Sirken, M. G. (1962): *J. nat. Cancer Inst., 28,* 947.

Haenzsel, W. and Kurihara, M. (1968): *J. nat. Cancer Inst., 40,* 43.

Henderson, B. E. et al. (1975): *Amer. J. Epidem. 101,* 477.

Higginson, J. and Muir, C. (1974): In: *Cancer Medicine.* Lea and Febiger, New York.

Hoover, R. and Fraumeni Jr., J. F. (1975): *Environ. Res., 9,* 196.

International Agency for Research on Cancer (1972-5): *Monographs on the Evaluation of Carcinogenic Risk of Chemicals to Man, Vols. 1-9.* Lyon.

Kuratsune, M. et al. (1974): *Int. J. Cancer, 13,* 552.

Langard, S. and Norseth, T. (1975): *Brit. J. industr. Med., 32,* 62.

Lloyd, J. W. (1971): *J. occup. Med., 13,* 53.

Mancuso, T. J. and Coulter, E. J. (1958): *J. nat. Cancer Inst., 20,* 79.

Mason, T. J. et al. (1975): *Atlas of Cancer Mortality for U.S. Counties, 1950-1969.* No. (NIH) 75-780. Bethesda, Md. U.S. Department of Health, Education and Welfare Publication.

Maugh, T. H. (1974): *Science, 186,* 1198.

McMichael, A. J., Spirtus, M. S., Kupper, L. L. and Gamble, J. F. (1975): *J. occup. Med., 17,* 234.

Menck, H. R., Casagrande, J. and Henderson, B. E. (1974): *Science, 183,* 210.

Milham, Jr, S. (1975): *J. occup. Med., 17,* 581.

Miller, R. W. (1969): In: *Abstracts, XVI International Congress on Occupational Health,* 233.

Office of Population Censuses and Surveys (1971): *Registrar-General's Decennial Supplement, England and Wales. Occupational Mortality Tables.* Her Majesty's Stationery Office, London.

Pedersen, E., Hogetreit, A. and Anderson, A. (1973): *Int. J. Cancer, 12,* 32.

Selikoff, I. J., Hammond, E. C. and Seidmen, H. (1973): In: *Biological Effects of Asbestos,* p. 209. International Agency for Research on Cancer, Lyon.

Spitzer, W. O. et al. (1975): *New Engl. J. Med.,* September.

Tomatis, L. (1975): In: *Proceedings, New York Academy of Science Conference on Occupational Carcinogenesis,* in press.

U.S. Department of Health, Education and Welfare (1963): *Mortality by Occupation and Cause of Death Among Men 20-44 Years of Age; U.S. 1950.* Vital Statistics Special Reports, U.S. Government Printing Office.

U.S. Department of Health, Education and Welfare (1967): *Occupational Characteristics of Disabled Workers by Disabling Conditions – Disability Insurance Benefit Awards made in 1959-62 to Men under age 65.* Public Health Service Publication No. 1530, Washington, D.C.

Persistent viral infections

David O. White

School of Microbiology, University of Melbourne, Parkville, Vic., Australia

As we enter the final quarter of the twentieth century vaccines have successively tamed smallpox, yellow fever, poliomyelitis, measles and rubella and the end is in sight for the last of the major acute viral diseases of man, hepatitis and influenza. The attention of virologists is turning towards a completely different class of disease, the existence of which was barely recognised until a few years ago. I refer to persistent viral infections, little known in man but well studied in animals, where they can manifest themselves as anything from insidious lethal disease of the brain to 'immune complex' or 'auto-immune' diseases and cancer. Such infections are variously referred to in the literature as 'latent', 'slow' or 'persistent', used virtually interchangeably. Fenner, Mims and I (Fenner et al., 1974; Fenner and White, 1976) have tried to introduce some order into this rather messy area of virology by defining three distinct types of persistent infection in terms of the characteristic behaviour of the virus in each instance (Fig. 1).

True latent infection is typified by herpes simplex or zoster. Following an acute infection, which may be clinical or subclinical, the virus persists in the body for a prolonged period, often for life, in a non-demonstrable form, until years later, in response to provocation such as irradiation or fever, the virus is

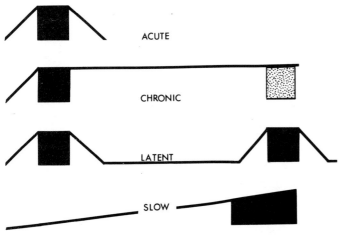

Fig. 1. Persistent viral infections. The solid line represents the concentration of virus in the body on a time scale measured in years. The solid boxes represent episodes of disease, whereas the stippled box indicates that disease sometimes develops as a late complication.

induced to multiply again. Such endogenous recrudescences of disease may recur.

A chronic infection may be defined as one in which the virus fails to be rejected following the initial infection and continues to be shed, often for years. Disease may be manifest only during the acute stages of the illness, or only as a late immunopathological or malignant complication of the viral carrier state.

A slow infection is one with a long incubation period attributable to very slow multiplication of virus which eventually leads to a progressive lethal disease.

Let us look at some human examples of each of these three major classes of persistent infection. The latent infection is perhaps the most familiar and is now widely recognised as the special province of the herpesviruses (Kaplan, 1974) (Table 1). Herpes simplex (Stevens and Cook, 1973) and varicella (Taylor-Robinson and Caunt, 1972) viruses take refuge in the neurons of the cerebral and spinal ganglia, where they persist for life in an occult form; they can be induced to multiply following prolonged in vitro cultivation of carrier ganglia.

Cytomegalovirus infection (Plummer, 1973; Weller, 1971) is common and usually inapparent except in the case of post-transfusion mononucleosis or cytomegalic inclusion disease, acquired transplacentally. Nevertheless, the virus can persist for years in B lymphocytes and can be reactivated by immunosuppression. A similar situation applies with the Epstein-Barr (EB) virus (Epstein

TABLE 1

Latent infections: virus non-demonstrable
between recrudescences

Virus	Carrier Cell
Herpes simplex	Neurons
Varicella-zoster	Neurons
Cytomegalovirus	Lymphocytes
EB virus	Lymphocytes

and Achong, 1973; Henle and Henle, 1972; Klein, 1972; Zur Hausen, 1972), a ubiquitous agent causing mononucleosis (glandular fever) in a minority of people and in most a subclinical infection which persists for life; the virus can be reactivated from normal lymphocytes by cultivation in vitro or treatment with bromodeoxyuridine. Immortal lymphoblastoid cell lines established from these cells resemble those of Burkitt's lymphoma which carry the EB virus genome, integrated into the chromosomes of the malignant cell. Despite the invariable association of EB virus with both Burkitt's lymphoma and the Chinese nasopharyngeal carcinoma, the etiological role of the virus, if any, has yet to be established. Undeniably, the attention of viral oncologists is focussing more sharply on the herpesviruses, particularly since the DNA of herpes simplex type 2 has been found to be integrated into the cells of most human cervical carcinomas (Nahmias and Roizman, 1973). If it transpires that herpesviruses are oncogenic for man, which they undoubtedly are for some other animals, it may be feasible to immunize against these cancers (Hilleman, 1973), as is already standard practice with Marek's disease of fowls (Purchase, 1974).

Chronic infections of man by viruses are not yet widely recognized (Table 2).

TABLE 2

Chronic infections: virus always demonstrable

Virus	Host	Disease
Hepatitis B	Man	Chronic hepatitis or nil
Rubella	Man	Rubella syndrome in fetus
LCM	Mouse	Immune complex disease
Aleutian disease	Mink	Immune complex disease
Infectious anemia	Horse	Immune complex disease
Leukemia	Mouse, chicken	Leukemia or nil

Perhaps the clearest example is hepatitis B (Blumberg et al., 1972; Purcell, 1975; *Amer. J. med. Sci.,* 1975; Vyas et al., 1972; World Health Organization, 1973; Zuckerman, 1975), in which the extraordinarily large numbers of virions and the associated HB-antigen (Australia antigen) demonstrable for years in the serum of some carriers constitute a real hazard to drug addicts, recipients of blood transfusions and the personnel of renal dialysis units. The rubella syndrome (Blattner et al., 1973; Catalano and Sever, 1971; Ciba Foundation, 1974; Fucillo and Sever, 1973; Rawls, 1974) can legitimately be regarded as a chronic infection of the fetus in which the virus continues to grow in clones of vital cells for up to several months after birth. We must turn to other animals for illustrative examples of the class of chronic infection characterized by the development late in life of a disease state attributable to the accumulation of virus-antibody complexes in glomeruli and arteries. Such 'immune complex disease' (Oldstone, 1975) is a conspicuous feature of lymphocytic choriomeningitis of mice (LCM) (Cole and Nathanson, 1974), Aleutian disease of mink (ADM) (Porter, 1974), lactate dehydrogenase-elevating (LDH) virus infection of mice (Riley, 1974) and equine infectious anemia (EIA) (Henson and McGuire, 1974). In all these infections the virus itself is non-cytocidal but for some reason fails to be neutralized by the very high levels of antibody that it induces, and eventually antigen-antibody complexes deposited in vital organs result in immune-complex disease. Similar pathology is seen in some cases of human viral hepatitis and we must ask how much of the idiopathic glomerulonephritis and how many of our so-called 'autoimmune' diseases may represent late consequences of a persistent viral infection. In the case of the leukemia viruses of mice, chickens, and now numerous other species, congenitally acquired infection is again completely harmless to the host, but later in life a proportion of the animals develop leukemia, possibly under the influence of some hormone or extrinsic 'carcinogen' of which we know nought (Baltimore, 1974; Emmelot and Bentvelzen, 1972; Gross, 1970; Hirsch and Black, 1974; McAllister, 1973; Silvestri, 1971; Temin, 1971; Todaro, 1973; Todaro and Huebner, 1972; Tooze, 1973; Wyke, 1974).

Slow virology (Brody et al., 1967; Fucillo et al., 1974; Gajdusek et al., 1965; Gajdusek and Gibbs, 1973; Hotchin, 1974; Porter, 1971; Zeman and Lennette, 1974) practised by slow virologists, bids fare to replace molecular virology as the glamour area of our discipline (Table 3). Kuru and Creutzfeldt-Jakob disease are rare fatal degenerative diseases of the human brain, known as subacute spongiform encephalopathies (Gajdusek and Gibbs, 1973) because of the characteristic slowly progressive vacuolation of neurons and proliferation and hypertrophy of astroglia leading to a spongiform appearance of the gray matter. Kuru (Gajdusek and Gibbs, 1973) is the only known disease considered to have been spread by cannibalism and is now virtually extinct; Creutzfeldt-Jakob disease is

TABLE 3

Slow infections: long incubation period; slowly fatal disease

Man		
Subacute sclerosing panencephalitis		Measles
Progressive multifocal leukoencephalopathy		Papovavirus
Kuru		Viroid?
Creutzfeldt-Jakob disease		Viroid?
Animals		
Visna-maedi	Sheep	Retrovirus
Scrapie	Sheep	Viroid?

a more cosmopolitan presenile dementia. Both are transmissible to primates, as is the agent of the prototype slow virus, scrapie of sheep, and it is now believed that all the spongiform encephalopathies may be caused by very similar agents, known in the trade as 'viroids'. Subacute sclerosing panencephalitis (Sever and Zeman, 1968; Ter Meulen et al., 1972) is a rare late complication of measles; the virus is present in the brain but can only be demonstrated following in vitro cultivation of the affected cells. Progressive multifocal leukoencephalopathy (Weiner et al., 1973; Zu Rhein, 1969) is seen only in very ill people whose immune system has been severely depressed by cancer or immunosuppressive therapy. Under these circumstances, the causative papovavirus, which sub-clinically infects most people, multiplies in oligodendrocytes and induces hyperplasia of astrocytes and demyelination of neurons. All four of these slow diseases of the human brain are very rare. The importance of the recent discoveries lies rather in the implication that more common diseases of the CNS, such as multiple sclerosis, Parkinson's disease or the more common presenile dementias may equally turn out to have a viral etiology.

Finally let me turn to the key question. Why is it that some acute viral infections fail to resolve? What is the basis of viral persistence? We can seek the answer in two directions. Do some viruses or viral mutants have unique properties that enable them to persist? Alternatively, are the immunological responses of some people inadequate to reject the virus? The answer is probably that persistent infections can arise in several different ways; indeed, there is evidence in the literature that leads us to this conclusion and I have tried to draw those threads together in Table 4.

The high priests of cancer virology have decreed that genetic information need no longer pass from DNA to RNA as enunciated in the dogma according to Jacob and Monod, but may forthwith flow from RNA to DNA through the

TABLE 4

Possible explanations of persistent infections

Integrated viral genome	Retroviruses, herpesviruses
Non-cytocidal virus	$\left\{\begin{array}{l}\text{Arenaviruses, rhabdoviruses} \\ \text{Paramyxoviruses, retroviruses}\end{array}\right.$
Temperature-sensitive mutant	Paramyxoviruses
Viroid (non-immunogenic)	Kuru, CJD, scrapie?
Non-neutralizing antibodies	LCM, LDH, EIA, ADM
Congenital ('tolerizing') infection	LCM, leukemia
Growth in macrophages	LCM, LDH, EIA, ADM
Immunosuppression	LCM, leukemia, ADM, CMV

medium of the magical 'reverse transcriptase' (Temin, 1971; Temin and Baltimore, 1972). This remarkable enzyme, present (by definition) in the virion of all 'retroviruses' (previously known as oncornaviruses), catalyses the transcription of a DNA copy of the viral RNA genome, and this copy is integrated into the genome of every cell of every mouse or chicken that has been properly examined. Very probably all cells of all mammals, including man, carry all the genetic information for one or more species of retrovirus, and this information is passed 'vertically' from one generation to the next as an integral part of the host's 'normal' DNA (Baltimore, 1974; Hirsch and Black, 1974; Temin, 1974; Todaro and Huebner, 1972; Tooze, 1973; Wyke, 1974). Only following exposure to irradiation or mutagenic chemicals is this information fully expressed and virions produced. Such retroviruses are not always oncogenic; indeed, some of them are xenotropic, i.e. cannot infect their own species. Some however are oncogenic and may be horizontally transmitted in nature to produce leukemias, sarcomas and carcinomas in a wide variety of mammalian and avian species. There is clear evidence that the DNA of most or all of the herpesviruses may persist in the cell genome in similar fashion (Biggs et al., 1972; Klein, 1972).

It is a striking coincidence that most, but not all, of the viruses with the property of establishing persistent infections in vivo or in vitro are relatively non-cytocidal even for cells in which they are growing productively. Cells producing arenaviruses, rhabdoviruses, retroviruses, and some paramyxoviruses go on dividing as if nothing had happened – viral production and cell division are in no way mutually exclusive (Choppin et al., 1971; Poste and Nicholson, 1975; Walker, 1968).

If one examines the strains of virus recoverable from persistent infections in vivo or in vitro (carrier cultures), one often finds them to be temperature-sensitive mutants of relatively low virulence. The full implications of this recent

TARGET   KILLER

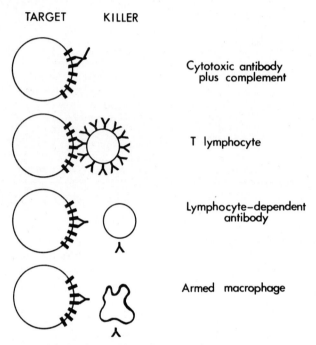

Cytotoxic antibody
plus complement

T lymphocyte

Lymphocyte–dependent
antibody

Armed macrophage

Fig. 2. Mechanisms of immune cytolysis of virus-infected cells. Virus-specific antigens in
the plasma membrane of infected cells may be the target for immunological attack by
specific antibody or antibody-bearing killer cells.

discovery have yet to be assessed, particularly in relation to the use of temperature-sensitive mutants as attenuated vaccines (Fenner, 1972; Wright et al., 1971).

The extraordinary agents responsible for the subacute spongiform encephalopathies do not resemble any known virus. They have not been seen and are not
neutralizable by antibody. The current view is that they may consist of a very
small molecule of nucleic acid protected by cellular membrane (Hunter, 1974). If
this is true, it is not difficult to envisage how such agents escape immune elimination by the body; it also raises fascinating questions about the mode of
replication and dissemination of these 'viroids' (Diener, 1974).

We come finally to a consideration of various types of immunological defects
(Allison, 1974; Blanden, 1974; Burns and Allison, 1975; Doherty and Zinkernagel, 1974; Mims, 1974; Notkins and Lodmell, 1975) that may enable even
perfectly immunogenic viruses to persist in vivo. Figure 2 summarises what one
surmises to be the four major mechanisms of immune cytolysis of virus-infected
cells.

Immune elimination of such infected cells, or indeed of virions themselves, can be blocked in vivo in a number of ways. Firstly, the very high titres of antibody elicited by infection with LCM, LDH, EIA or ADM seem to be non-neutralizing; in fact, it is the accumulation of the virus-antibody complexes in the body that eventually causes the characteristic immune-complex disease. Furthermore these complexes may block immune cytolysis of virus-infected target cells by immune T lymphocytes. In the case of certain congenitally acquired viruses the host may be, at least partially, tolerant to the virus and never succeed in mounting a really satisfactory immune response. Many of the viruses mentioned also grow in macrophages and destroy them (Allison, 1974). By this and/or other means they succeed in depressing the immune responses of the host.

This has been, by necessity, no more than a quick reconnoitre of the largely uncharted ocean of persistent viral infections. We have dared to plumb the dark waters in search of mechanisms, but have scarcely left a ripple on the surface.

References

Allison, A. C. (1974): *Transplant. Rev., 19,* 3.

American Journal of Medical Science (1975): Symposium on viral hepatitis. In Press.

Baltimore, D. (1974): *Cold Spr. Harb. Symp. quant. Biol., 39.*

Biggs, P. M., De Thé, G. and Payne, L. N. (ed.) (1972): *Oncogenesis and Herpesviruses.* Cancer Research Publication No. 2. International Agency for Research on Cancer, Lyon.

Blanden, R. V. (1974): *Transplant. Rev., 19,* 56.

Blattner, R. J., Williamson, A. P. and Heys, F. M. (1973): *Progr. med. Virol., 15,* 1.

Blumberg, B. S., Sutnick, A. I., London, W. T. and Millman I. (1972): *Australia Antigen and Hepatitis.* Chemical Rubber Co. Press, Cleveland.

Brody, J. A., Henle, W. and Koprowski, H. (ed.) (1967): *Curr. Top. Microbiol. Immunol., 40,* 1.

Burns, W. H. and Allison, A. C. (1975): *Advanc. Virus Res., 20,* in press.

Catalano, L. W. and Sever, J. L. (1971): *Ann. Rev. Microbiol., 25,* 255.

Choppin, P. W., Klenk, H. D., Compans, R. W. and Caliguiri, L. A. (1971): *Perspect. Virol., 7,* 127.

Ciba Foundation (1974): *Intrauterine Infections.* Ciba Foundation Symposia No. 10 (new series). Associated Scientific Publishers, Amsterdam.

Cole, G. A. and Nathanson, N. (1974): *Progr. med. Virol., 18,* 94.

Diener, T. O. (1974): *Ann. Rev. Microbiol., 28,* 23.

Doherty, P. C. and Zinkernagel, R. M. (1974): *Transplant Rev., 19,* 89.

Emmelot, P. and Bentvelzen, P. (ed.) (1972): *RNA viruses and Host Genome in Oncogenesis.* North-Holland Publishing Co., Amsterdam.

Epstein, M. A. and Achong, B. G. (1973): *Ann. Rev. Microbiol., 27,* 413.

Fenner, F. (1972): In: *Immunity in Viral and Rickettsial Diseases*, p. 131. Editors: A. Kohn and M. A. Klingberg. Plenum Press, New York.

Fenner, F., McAuslan, B. R., Mims, C. A., Sambrook, J. F. and White, D. O. (1974): *The Biology of Animal Viruses*, 2nd ed. Academic Press, New York.

Fenner, F. and White, D. O. (1976): *Medical Virology*, 2nd ed. Academic Press, New York.

Fuccillo, D. A., Kurent, J. E. and Sever, J. L. (1974): *Ann. Rev. Microbiol., 28,* 231.

Fucillo, D. A. and Sever, J. L. (1973): *Bact. Rev., 37,* 19.

Gajdusek, D. C. and Gibbs, Jr, C. J. (1973): *Perspect. Virol., 8,* 279.

Gajdusek, D. C., Gibbs C. J. and Alpers, M. (1965): *Slow, Latent and Temperate Virus Infections.* National Institute for Neurological Diseases Blindness Monograph No. 2. U.S. Government Printing Office, Washington, D.C.

Gross, L. (1970): *Oncogenic Viruses*, 2nd ed. Pergamon Press, Oxford.

Henle, W. and Henle, G. (1972): In: *Oncogenesis and Herpesviruses.* Editors: P. M. Biggs, G. de Thé and L. N. Payne. Cancer Research Publications No. 2. International Agency for Research on Cancer, Lyon.

Henson, J. B. and McGuire, T. C. (1974): *Progr. med. Virol., 18,* 143.

Hilleman, M. R. (1973): *Perspect. Virol., 8,* 119.

Hirsch, M. S. and Black, P. H. (1974): *Advanc. Virus Res., 19,* 265.

Hotchin, J. (ed.) (1974): *Progr. med. Virol., 18.*

Hunter, G. D. (1974): *Progr. med. Virol., 18,* 289.

Kaplan, A. S. (ed.) (1974): *The Herpesviruses.* Academic Press, New York.

Klein, G. (1972): *Proc. nat. Acad. Sci. (Wash.), 69,* 1056.

McAllister, R. M. (1973): *Progr. med. Virol., 16,* 48.

Mims, C. (1974): *Progr. med. Virol., 18,* 1.

Nahmias, A. J. and Roizman, B. (1973): *New Engl. J. Med., 289,* 667, 719, 781.

Notkins, A. L. and Lodmell, J. (1975): *Perspect. Virol.,* in press.

Oldstone, M. B. A. (1975): *Progr. med. Virol., 19,* 84.

Plummer, G. (1973): *Progr. med. Virol., 15,* 92.

Porter, D. D. (1974): *Progr. med. Virol., 18,* 32.

Porter, D. D. (1971): *Progr. med. Virol., 13,* 339.

Poste, G. and Nicholson, G. (ed.) (1975): *Virus Infections and the Cell Surface.* North Holland Publishing Co., Amsterdam.

Purcell, R. H. (1975): *Perspect. Virol., 9,* in press.

Purchase, H. G. (1974): *Progr. med. Virol., 18,* 179.

Rawls, W. E. (1974): *Progr. med. Virol., 18,* 273.

Riley, V. (1974): *Progr. med. Virol., 18,* 199.

Sever, J. L. and Zeman, W. (ed.) (1968): *Neurology (Minneap.), 18,* Part 2.

Silvestri, L. G. (ed.) (1971): *The Biology of Oncogenic Viruses.* North-Holland Publishing Co., Amsterdam.

Stevens, J. G. and Cook, M. L. (1973): *Perspect. Virol., 8,* 171.

Taylor-Robinson, D. and Caunt, A. E. (1972): *Virol. Monogr., 12.*

Temin, H. M. (1971): *Ann. Rev. Microbiol., 25,* 609.

Temin, H. M. (1974): *Ann. Rev. Genet., 8,* 155.

Temin, H. M. and Baltimore, D. (1972): *Advanc. Virus Res., 17,* 129.

Ter Meulen, V., Katz, M. and Müller, D. (1972): *Curr. Top. Microbiol. Immunol., 57,* 1.

Todaro, G. J. (1973): *Perspect. Virol., 8,* 81.

Todaro, G. J. and Huebner, R. J. (1972): *Proc. nat. Acad. Sci. (Wash.), 69,* 1009.

Tooze, J. (1974): *Cold Spr. Harb. Symp. quant. Biol., 39.*

Vyas, G. N., Perkins, H. A. and Schmid, R. (ed.) (1972): *Hepatitis and Blood Transfusion.* Grune and Stratton, New York.

Walker, D. L. (1968): In: *Medical and Applied Virology,* p. 99. Editors: M. Sanders and E. H. Lennette. W. Green, St. Louis.

Weiner, L. P., Johnson, R. T. and Herndon, R. M. (1973): *New Engl. J. Med., 288,* 1103.

Weller, T. H. (1971): *New Engl. J. Med., 285,* 203 and 267.

World Health Organization (1973): *Wld. Hlth. Org. techn. Rep. Ser., 512.*

Wright, P. F., Mills, J. and Chanock, R. M. (1971). *J. infect. Dis., 124,* 505.

Wyke, J. A. (1974): *Int. Rev. Cytol., 38,* 68.

Zeman, W. and Lennette, E. J. (ed.) (1974): *Slow Virus Diseases.* Williams and Wilkins, Baltimore.

Zuckerman, A. J. (1975): *Human Viral Hepatitis: Hepatitis-Associated Antigen and Viruses.* 2nd ed. North-Holland Publishing Co., Amsterdam.

Zur Hausen, H. (1972): *Int. Rev. exp. Path., 11,* 233.

Zu Rhein, G. M. (1969): *Progr. med. Virol., 11,* 185.

5: The nature of tumours

The pathogenesis of neoplasia in man

*Department of Medical Oncology, Imperial Cancer Research Fund,
St. Bartholomew's Hospital, London, U.K.*

There are many changes, both morphological and functional, both in vitro and in vivo, which occur in malignant cells in man. However, which of all these are responsible for conferring on a cell the biological properties of malignancy is uncertain. Only a few can be considered, including:

1. The development of tumour-associated antigens (the biologically important ones in transplantation experiments in animals being individually specific in chemically induced tumours, but group-specific in those caused by viruses) and the significance of their release into the circulation.

2. The development of antibodies, not only to tumour-associated antigens, but also to a wide range of normal tissues such as DNA and smooth muscle.

---

* *Editorial Note:* It was with deepest regret that the Scientific Programme Committee learned of the tragic death of Professor Gordon Hamilton Fairley which occurred almost as soon as he returned to London from Congress. Professor Fairley's Address to Congress was as usual brilliant in content and presentation and delivered largely from slides without formal text. Unfortunately, the only material now available for publication is this summary which was submitted before the meeting. E.S.F.

3. The release into the circulation of substances which can be detected (a) by chemical means such as alpha-foetoprotein in hepatocellular carcinoma and immunoglobulin or its subunits with myelomatosis and macroglobulinaemia, (b) by their endocrine function such as human chorionic gonadotrophin in choriocarcinoma, erythropoietin in renal tumours, and rarely in other tumours, and inappropriate anti-diuretic hormone in carcinoma of the bronchus, etc., and (c) by immunological techniques such as the detection of carcinoembryonic antigen in various forms of malignancy as well as some benign diseases.

4. The induction of malignant change in benign cells as illustrated by the patient described by Thomas et al. (1972), in whom a relapse of acute leukaemia occurred in the donor cells following a marrow graft.

The significance of these and other changes, particularly those involving chromosomal abnormalities and DNA, will be discussed in relation to the current theories of the pathogenesis of the malignant change, and in particular in relation to the clonal theory of malignancy (Burnet, 1972).

References

Burnet, F. M. (1972): *Autoimmunity and Autoimmune Disease.* Medical and Technical Publishing Co. Limited, London.
Thomas, E. D., Bryant, J. I., Buckner, O. D., Clift, R. A., Fefer, A., Johnson, F. L., Neiman, P., Ramberg, R. E. and Storb, R. (1972): *Lancet, 1,* 1310.

The interrelationship of lymphoreticular hyperplasia and neoplasia*

A. H. T. Robb-Smith

Radcliffe Infirmary, Oxford, U.K.

In view of the theme of this congress, it seemed appropriate to discuss the emergence of malignancy from reactive proliferation, which is a general biological phenomenon that is particularly well displayed in lymphoreticular tissue. Though recognised some sixty years ago, it has been much neglected, owing to the popularity of the hold-all concept of malignant lymphoma, which, as even its originator, Theodor Billroth (1871), admitted over a century ago, was extremely difficult to define pathologically or clinically and had little merit except as a collective term.

In 1913 Adami suggested that it would be desirable to distinguish from true neoplasms a group of diffuse overgrowths, for which he proposed the unhappy term 'hyperblastosis'; these might be regarded as due to a disturbance of metabolic equilibrium, and (with considerable prescience) he continued might 'possibly be combated eventually (certainly not today) along the lines of organotherapy' (Adami, 1918). He concluded by saying 'every transition is observable in this

---

* This invited paper was given following Plenary Session 5 among the Proffered Papers on histopathology.

series between the development of overgrowths of fully differentiated tissue, non-malignant grades of anaplasia and diffuse malignant infiltrative growths'.

Ewing (1928) endorsed this viewpoint and suggested that in considering lymphoid disorders one had to recognise various processes, some of which were inflammatory, some neoplastic and others intermediate in position, and he characterised certain tumour-like hyperplasias of lymphoid tissue. Warthin (1931) was the advocate of the concept of 'lymphoblastoma' as a term to cover the leukaemias, Hodgkin's disease and mycosis fungoides etc., all of which were neoplasms; there were transitional forms between them and one might be transformed into another.

It was Pullinger (1932) who, in a masterly study of Hodgkin's disease which is all too little known, adopted Letterer's (1924) term 'reticulosis', a collective title for the group of progressive hyperplasias. A little later, Theodore Waugh (1937), an associate of Oertel at McGill, in an admirable paper on the interrelation of various systemic haematopoietic processes, set out clearly which conditions he would regard as hyperplastic, which neoplastic and which intermediate, though for this group he put forward the etymologically unreasonable term 'kataplasia', which is sometimes to be found in the Japanese writings (Tanaka, 1973).

I think it is important to emphasise that these writers were not solely concerned with a biological concept, but took the view that one could distinguish individual lymphoid disorders with a characteristic histology and natural history, in opposition to the malignant lymphoma school, which believed in a striking fluidity in the histological pattern of lymphoid conditions with transitions and combinations between them, but had little interest in attempts to identify clinicopathological entities.

The death knell of the fluid lymphoma school was probably first heard at the American Society of Clinical Pathology seminar in 1958 when Gall and Rappaport (1958), after three years of what they described as 'fiery debate and negotiation', introduced a classification of malignant lymphoma segregated both as to cell type and whether it was nodular or diffuse, but, even more significant, at this seminar, the interlocutors were prepared to recognise nine distinct types of primary lymphadenopathy, eight reactive lymphadenopathies as well as storage disorders and metastatic growths. Five years later Lukes (1963) presented his first paper on the types of Hodgkin's disease in relation to prognosis, which ten years ago was transformed in upper New York State into the Rye classification (Lukes, 1966). The following year, the Lymphology Congress at Zurich had presentations on the European and American classification of malignant lymphoma by Lennert (1967) and Lukes (1967). Lennert recognised the three categories of lymphadenopathies – reactive, sarcomatous, and an intermediate group which he designated 'autonomous hyperplasia' and which embraced a wide range of conditions – whereas Lukes, who admitted that 'though the majority of United States pathologists generally agree on the definition of malignant lymphoma as a malignant neoplasm of lymph node derivatives, beyond that there is no agreement', followed Gall and Rappaport very closely, though stressing the importance of blood and plasma protein changes. The joint U.S.-Japanese meetings in 1967 and 1971 revealed that the Japanese pathologists not only recognised the morphological character of progressive hyperplasia (Iijima, 1973; Sucha and Ota, 1973) but also adopted the viewpoint that the sarcomas of lymphoreticular tissue, reticulosarcomata – which might or might not embrace the lymphosarcomata – had all the attributes of a typical malignant neoplasm (Akazaki, 1973). It was at these meetings that Kojima et al. (1973), Lennert (1973) and Lukes and Collins (1973) first put forward their views that the follicular lymphoma was derived from the cells of the germinal centre and so introduced the concept of immunotopography into lymph node pathology (Robb-Smith, 1974) and it is certain that it was the work of Nossal et al. (1968) that initiated this new dynamic approach. It was Jones et al. (1972) who introduced the term 'non-Hodgkin's lymphoma' for the group of conditions included in the classification put forward by Rappaport in 1966, and this term was adopted for the title of an excellent symposium held in London (Peckham, 1975), which embraced a far wider range of lymph node topics. Last year we were subjected to a plague of non-Hodgkin's lymphoma classifications which was silenced by the witty intervention of Kay (1974). The only significant one was the Kiel classification (Gérard-Marchant et al., 1974) on which Lennert et al. (1975) provided an admirable gloss at the International Congress of Haematology in London this summer. The Kiel classification distinguishes malignant lymphomas of low- and high-grade malignancy, each of which are subdivided according to the predominant cell type, and the cytological descriptions and illustrations should enable identification in most cases, irrespective of the nomenclature employed. It is stated that the low-grade malignant lymphomas correspond to the progressive hyperplasia (reticulosis) of Robb-Smith (1938, 1964) and embrace chronic lymphatic leukaemia (both B and T cell type), hairy cell leukaemia, Sézary's syndrome and mycosis fungoides, Waldenstrom's macroglobulinaemia, lymphocytic lymphosarcoma and follicular lymphoma, while the high-grade malignant group includes the Burkitt tumour, lymphoblastic sarcoma, etc.

It would be undesirable to get involved in the problem of nomenclature of lymph node disorders and cytology, as far too many pathologists have adopted the Humpty Dumpty etymological principle ('When I use a word, it means just what I choose it to mean, neither more nor less'), but we do well to recall that 'reticulosis' (Letterer, 1924; Tchistowitch and Bykowa, 1928; Oberling and Guerin, 1934; Pullinger, 1932; Ross, 1933; Robb-Smith, 1938) and 'reticulosarcoma' (Oberling, 1928), when introduced over a quarter of a century ago, were collective terms to embrace a whole range of progressive hyperplasias and neoplasms. They were based on Maximow's concept that the undifferentiated reticulum cell was a pluripotential cell which could differentiate along haemic (lymphoid, myeloid, monocytic), phagocytic (histiocyte littoral cells) and fibrocytic lines; whether such a cell type can be identified in post-embryonic life may be in doubt, but from the point of view of descriptive morphology the concept is certainly convenient. It was long after this that the term 'reticulum cell sarcoma' was used to describe a poorly differentiated malignant neoplasm thought to be of histiocytic origin (Gall and Mallory, 1942), but electron microscopy and immunohistology have shown that tumours having, under the light microscope, the features believed to indicate a histiocytic origin are more probably of a lymphoid nature.

The recent spate of classifications, often described as functional, have paid scant attention to the natural history or the clinical features of the various cytological types which have been segregated. Any critical histologist studying lymph node disorders would be aware that a proliferation could take place in the follicles, the sinuses or the interfollicular area (now known as the paracortical or T cell area). It would also be apparent that if there was a proliferation in one compartment, when generalised it would be mirrored in other organs: for example, a follicular proliferation in lymph nodes would also involve the malpighian bodies of the spleen and there would be follicle-like proliferations in the periportal tissue, bone marrow, dermis, etc. We now know that the majority of the follicular cells are B or bursa-equivalent and that the phenomenon of homing or ecotaxis (De Sousa, 1971) may be a consequence of differences in the cell surface of B and T lymphocytes. However there is little evidence of disturbance of antibody function associated with B-type lymphadenopathies or of cell-mediated immunity with T cell disorders, and their functional characters are very varied. For example there is good evidence that both Sézary's syndrome and Sternberg's 'leukosarcoma' are of T cell origin, yet one is a relatively benign condition in the elderly initially involving the dermis, while the other is a highly malignant mediastinal neoplasm in teenagers, though in both conditions the abnormal cells are to be found in the circulating blood.

I am not suggesting that immunotopographical studies of lymphoreticular disorders are undesirable. Far from it, but I think that this new knowledge should be applied in attempts to provide increased precision in prognosis and response to treatment rather than to the creation of philosophical systems.

Returning to the relationship between progressive hyperplasia and truly malignant neoplasms, we may consider one or two examples quite briefly.

Follicular lymphoma is essentially a disorder of the fifth and sixth decades which causes relatively little inconvenience and, provided the patients are not over-treated, has little influence on life expectancy, but in about 20% of all cases, after this comparatively benign course has proceeded for ten or so years, there is a sudden change, with rapid enlargement of nodes and extra nodal masses, which become relatively radioresistant, and the patients succumb in a matter of months. Instead of the well patterned follicles of cleaved cells there is a disruption of follicles, a change in cell type to a more poorly differentiated form, infiltration, with stromal destruction and extra nodal metastases. This is an excellent example of sarcomatous change from a progressive hyperplasia (Robb-Smith, 1947; Spiro et al., 1975).

Much less common is sarcomatous change in lymphocytic preponderant Hodgkin's disease (Robb-Smith, 1947), myeloma (Holt and Robb-Smith, 1973), chronic myeloid leukaemia (Suchi and Ota, 1973). Inevitably the question must arise as to whether therapy had induced the sarcomatous change or whether the increased survival consequent on improved therapy had allowed the change to develop; on the whole the evidence would favour the former hypothesis. It is also necessary to consider the possibility that persistent antigenic stimulation may induce a reactive hyperplasia which will become a progressive hyperplasia and ultimately result in a reticulosarcoma. Probably the most detailed studies have been made in relation to lymphadenopathy complicating idiopathic steatorrhoea (Whitehead, 1968) and again the interval between symptoms of steatorrhoea and development of sarcoma is about ten years. The sarcoma is in fact a histiocytic reticulosarcoma. Seligmann (1975) has described the progression from a reactive change to a sarcoma in alpha chain disease. Then there is the association of holoendemic malaria, big spleen disease and histiocytic medullary reticulosis which has been described in Uganda. The development of progressive hyperplasia and sometimes sarcoma in Sjögren's disease, congenital immune deficiencies and a chronic immunosuppression are all examples of this interrelationship, and finally there is the development of progressive hyperplasia and sarcoma in certain strains of mice (NZB, SJL/J, PBA and chronic allogeneic disease) which Taylor (1974), working in my department, has studied. He has been able to show that initially there is a reactive hyperplasia with plasma cell proliferation which leads to a progressive hyperplasia and ultimately a sarcoma which is derived from B lymphocytes. The experimental evidence which he and others have produced would suggest that the persistent antigenic stimulation provides an environment in which the target cells are susceptible to an oncogenic virus.

It would be inexpedient to translate the results of animal experimentation to human disease, but there is clearly an analogy and it would be more easily recognised and studied if the concept of progressive hyperplasia of lymphoid tissue which could lead to sarcomatous change was more widely recognised.

References

Adami, J. G. (1918): *Medical Contributions to the Study of Evolution*, p. 340. Macmillan, London.

Akazaki, K. (1973): In: *Gann Monograph on Cancer Research No. 15*, p. 21. Editors: K. Akazaki, H. Rappaport, C. W. Berard, J. M. Bennett and E. Ishikawa. Japanese Cancer Association.

Billroth, T. (1871): *Wien. med. Wschr.*, 1065.

De Sousa, (1971): *Clin. exp. Immunol., 9*, 371.

Ewing, J. (1928): *Neoplastic Diseases, 3rd ed.* (1940, 4th ed.). W. B. Saunders, Philadelphia.

Gérard-Marchant, R., Hamlin, I., Lennert, K., Rilke, F., Stanfield, A. G. and Van Unnik, J. A. M. (1974): *Lancet, 2,* 406.

Gall, E. A. and Mallory, T. B. (1942): *Amer. J. Path., 18,* 381.

Gall, E. A. and Rappaport, H. (1958): In: *Proceedings, 23rd Seminar on Diseases of Lymph Nodes and Spleen*, p. 107. Editor: McDonald. American Society of Clinical Pathologists.

Holt, J. M. and Robb-Smith, A. H. T. (1973): *J. clin. Path., 26,* 649.

Iijima, S. (1973): In: *Gann Monograph on Cancer Research No. 15*, p. 163. Editors: K. Akazaki, H. Rappaport, C. W. Berard, J. M. Bennett and E. Ishikawa. Japanese Cancer Association.

Jones, G. E., Kaplan, H. S. and Rosenberg, S. A. (1972): *Cancer (Philad.), 29,* 954.

Kay, A. E. M. (1974): *Lancet, 2,* 586.

Kojima, M., Imai, Y. and Mori, N. (1973): In: *Gann Monograph on Cancer Research No. 15,* p. 195. Editors: K. Akazaki, H. Rappaport, C. W. Berard, J. M. Bennett and E. Ishikawa. Japanese Cancer Association.

Lennert, K. (1967): In: *Progress in Lymphology*, p. 103. Editor: A. Rüttimann. G. Thieme, Stuttgart.

Lennert, K. (1973): In: *Gann Monographs on Cancer Research* No. 15, p. 217. Editors: K. Akazaki, H. Rappaport, C. W. Berard, J. M. Bennett and E. Ishikawa. Japanese Cancer Association.

Lennert, K., Mohri, N., Stein, H. and Kaisorling, E. (1975): *Brit. J. Haemat., 31, Suppl. 143.*

Letterer, E. (1924): *Frankfurt. Z. Path., 30,* 377.

Lukes, R. J. (1963): *Amer. J. Roentgenol., 90,* 944.

Lukes, R. J. (1966): *Cancer Res., 26.*

Lukes, R. J. (1967): In: *Progress in Lymphology*, p. 109. Editor: A. Rüttimann. G. Thieme, Stuttgart.

Lukes, R. J. and Collins, R. D. (1973): In: *Gann Monograph on Cancer Research No. 15,* p. 209. Editors: K. Akazaki, H. Rappaport, C. W. Berard, J. M. Bennett and E. Ishikawa. Japanese Cancer Association.

Nossal, G. J. V., Abbot, A., Mitchell, J. and Lummus, Z. (1968): *J. exp. med., 127,* 277.

Oberling, C. (1928): *Bull. Ass. franç. Cancer., 17,* 259.

Oberling, C. and Guerin, M. (1934): *Sang, 8,* 892.

Peckham, B. (ed.) (1975): *Brit. J. Cancer, Suppl. 11.*

Pullinger, B. (1932): *Research on Lymphadenoma.* John Wright, Bristol.

Rappaport, H. (1966): In: *Atlas of Tumour Pathology,* Section III, Fascicle 8. Armed Forces Institute of Pathology, Washington, D.C.

Robb-Smith, A. H. T. (1938): *J. Path. Bact., 47,* 457.

Robb-Smith, A. H. T. (1947): In: *Recent Advances in Clinical Pathology.* Editor: S. C. Dyke. Churchill, London.

Robb-Smith, A. H. T. (1964): In: *Treatment of Cancer and Allied Diseases,* Vol. 9, p. 1. Editors: G. T. Park and I. M. Ariel. Hoeber Medical Division, Harper and Row, New York.

Robb-Smith, A. H. T. (1974): *Lancet, 1,* 513.

Ross, J. (1933): *J. Path. Bact., 37,* 311.

Seligmann, M. (1975): *Brit. J. Cancer, 31, Suppl. II,* 356.

Spiro, G., Galton, D. A. G., Wiltshaw, E. and Lohman, R. C. (1975): *Brit. J. Cancer, 31, Suppl. II,* 60.

Suchi, T. and Ota, K. (1973): In: *Gann Monograph on Cancer Research No. 15,* p. 97. Editors: K. Akazaki, H. Rappaport, G. W. Berard, J. M. Bennett and E. Ishikawa. Japanese Cancer Association.

Tanaka, N. (1973): In: *Gann Monograph on Cancer Research No. 15,* p. 123. Editors: K. Akazaki, H. Rappaport, C. W. Berard, J. M. Bennett and E. Ishikawa. Japanese Cancer Association.

Taylor, C. (1974): *An Immuno-Histological Study of Human and Murine Lymphomata.* D. Phil. thesis, University of Oxford.

Tchistowitch, K. and Bykowa, L. (1928): *Virchows Arch. path. Anat., 267,* 91.

Warthin, A. S. (1931): *Ann. Surg., 93,* 153.

Waugh, T. R. (1937): *Amer. J. med. Sci., 193,* 337.

Whitehead, R. (1968): *Gut, 9,* 569.

6: The behaviour of tumours

Unusual manifestations of cancer*

Sheldon C. Sommers

Department of Pathology, Lenox Hill Hospital, New York, N.Y., U.S.A.

Growth is an ordinary aspect of both normal organisms and neoplasms. The characteristic invasive and metastasizing attributes of cancer likewise are shared by normal trophoblastic cells, megakaryocytes and perhaps endometriosis. Among the many unusual properties of neoplasms, greater attention has recently been focused on ectopic hormone secretion.

Particularly pulmonary oat cell carcinomas, certain thymomas and pancreatic islet carcinomas may produce unexpected polypeptide hormones. These and other related cells are unified under Pearse's APUD endocrine system of neuroendocrine embryology and activity (Pearse, 1974). By histochemical and electron microscopic studies typical neuroendocrine granules are identified.

The kinds of polypeptide hormones produced by such APUDomas are unusual, since macromolecular forms such as big ACTH, big big ACTH, big gastrin and others are identified by plasma radioimmunoassay (Gewirtz and Yalow, 1974). In normal endocrine cells the larger prohormones are trypsinized in the cytoplasm and secreted as classical ACTH, gastrin, insulin, etc. (Lacy, 1975; Walsh and Grossman, 1975).

---

* Aided by grants from the Council for Tobacco U.S.A., Inc.

Dysplastic bronchial epithelial neuroendocrine cells have been reported to secrete big ACTH (Gewirtz and Yalow, 1974). Our current investigation of electron micrographs of dysplastic and normal human bronchial neuroendocrine epithelial cells (Terzakis et al., 1972) has uncovered two statistically significant differences in their organelle ultrastructure which are believed relevant to the size of the hormone molecules produced: (1) Golgi vesicles are smaller ($P < 0.01$) and (2) secretory granules are fewer ($P < 0.05$) in dysplastic than in normal bronchial neuroendocrine cells. Comparable defects were also observed in pulmonary oat cell and pancreatic islet carcinomas so far studied. It appears that macromolecular peptide hormones such as big ACTH or big gastrin are secreted ectopically from some dysplastic and neoplastic neuroendocrine cells partly because of underdeveloped Golgi vesicles in which the trypsinization of prohormones may normally occur.

Material and methods

Electron micrographs previously made as part of a study of human bronchial changes with aging were reviewed. Two groups were analyzed: (1) ten cases with bronchial dysplasia found by light microscopy in uninvolved segmental bronchi of surgical or autopsy specimens of lung carcinomas; (2) eight cases with histologically normal segmental bronchi, matched by age and sex for the prior aging study. Neuroendocrine bronchial epithelial cells were all scrutinized for quantitative changes in the following organelles: Golgi vesicles sizes and numbers; Golgi cisternae diameters; secretory granules sizes and numbers; relation of secretory granules to organelle and cell wall membranes (Palade, 1975).

The features enumerated were evaluated by measuring their sizes on photographic prints, or counting the items as appropriate. Means and standard deviations were calculated. Statistical t tests were utilized and revealed no significant differences between the dysplastic and normal groups, perhaps because of large differences in the standard deviations. Nonparametric Mann-Whitney rank tests were thereafter applied (Snedecor and Cochran, 1967).

Results

Dysplastic neuroendocrine bronchial epithelial cells had significantly smaller Golgi vesicles than the comparable normal cells ($P < 0.01$). Golgi cisternae, the sizes of secretory granules, and the relations of secretory granules to internal and external cell membranes showed no differences between the two groups. However, there were significantly fewer secretory granules in dysplastic than in normal neurosecretory bronchial cells (P < 0.05).

Discussion

This study attempts to provide a morphologic correlate for the observation of Gewirtz and Yalow (1974) that dysplastic and neoplastic bronchial epithelial cells secrete macromolecular forms of ACTH, called big ACTH and big big ACTH.

According to Lacy (1975), in pancreatic islet and other endocrine cells the cytoplasmic prohormones initially formed are larger molecules than those eventually secreted. Within the endocrine cell, at an undetermined site, the prohormone is normally trypsinized into subunits of conventional hormone molecular size, which are then stored and thereafter secreted into the blood. The present study points to the shrunken Golgi vesicles as a possible site where there is defective trypsinization of macromolecular prohormone of ACTH. The resulting fewer secretory granules per cell, and inferentially storage within them of the prohormone, appear to represent correlated observations.

Little quantitative ultrastructural analysis of Golgi apparatuses has been published. Sturgess and Moscarello (1975) have found that rat hepatocytic Golgi apparatuses become hypertrophied after recent exposure to hepatotoxins. Golgi atrophy in rats followed either protein starvation or perturbation following puromycin administration.

In our initial ultrastructural studies of pulmonary oat cell carcinoma, medullary thyroid carcinoma and pancreatic islet cell carcinoma, it appears that their cells too possess shrunken Golgi vesicles and fewer secretory granules, as compared to their normal cellular counterparts. Collection of adequate numbers of cases for the statistical analysis of measurements of various organelles will now be necessary.

Meanwhile from these and other data it is possible to see a field of quantitative ultrastructural pathology emerging. Normal, dysplastic and neoplastic cells are recognized as being responsive to internal and external environmental influences.

Summary

Compared to the normal human bronchial neuroendocrine epithelial cells, dysplastic epithelial cells had smaller Golgi vesicles and fewer secretory gra-

nules. These ultrastructural differences may correlate with the preferential secretion of big ACTH by dysplastic and neoplastic pulmonary epithelium. Some
pulmonary oat cell carcinomas, medullary thyroid carcinomas and pancreatic
islet carcinomas appear to share these ultrastructural abnormalities.

References

Gewirtz, B. and Yalow, R. S. (1974): *J. clin. Invest., 53,* 1022.
Lacy, P. (1975): *Amer. J. Path., 79,* 170.
Palade, G. (1975): *Science, 189,* 347.
Pearse, A. G. E. (1974): *Path. Ann., 9,* 27.
Snedecor, G. W. and Cochran, W. G. (1967): *Statistical Methods,* p. 130. Iowa State
    University Press, Ames, Iowa.
Sturgess, J. M. and Moscarello, M. A. (1975): *Pathobiol. Ann.,* in press.
Terzakis, J. A., Sommers, S. C. and Andersson, B. (1972): *Lab. Invest., 26,* 127.
Walsh, J. H. and Grossman, M. I. (1975): *New Engl. J. Med., 292,* 1324.

Immunological control of cancer*

D. S. Nelson

Kolling Institute of Medical Research,
The Royal North Shore Hospital of Sydney,
St. Leonards, New South Wales, Australia

The development and growth of a malignant tumour are accompanied by extensive immunological activities. Most tumours – probably all – possess antigens which the normal immune system recognizes and against which it reacts. There is evidence that the normally functioning immune system is mostly successful in exercising surveillance over the emergence of altered, potentially malignant cells, so that the establishment of a primary tumour represents a failure of the immune system. There is also increasing evidence that interactions between the immune system and tumour antigens can have secondary effects on the host, and that some tumours may release substances which non-specifically depress host

* The work of the author's laboratory is supported in part by grants from the New South Wales State Cancer Council, the National Health and Medical Research Council, the Australian Kidney Foundation and the Postgraduate Medical Foundation of The University of Sydney. Some is carried out pursuant to Research Contract NO1-CB-63973 with the National Cancer Institute, United States Department of Health, Education and Welfare.

immunity. Furthermore, interactions of host with tumour are chronic processes occurring over a far longer period of time than with any except the most chronic of microbial infections. It has been estimated that a palpable breast cancer nodule, about 1 cm in diameter, may have taken between eight and forty years to develop (Bond, 1968, quoted by Lindenmann, 1974). Distant metastases may not manifest themselves for five to ten years, if at all, after tumour cells have been demonstrated in the circulation at the time of 'definitive' surgical treatment of a primary tumour (Roberts et al., 1967; Smith, 1972). Cancer may, indeed, be clinically apparent for only a brief part of the natural history of the disease.

The phrase 'immunological control of cancer' can have a variety of meanings. It is convenient to examine the ways in which control can be exerted in relation to different stages in the natural history of cancer.

It is almost instinctive for immunologists to seek to prevent a disease by means of immunization or vaccination. In relation to human cancer one can contemplate immunoprophylaxis in two ways: the use of vaccines to prevent or abort infection with oncogenic viruses, or the use of non-specific immunopotentiating agents to raise the general level of immunocompetence or, in other words, to step up the surveillance. Reasons for scepticism about the general value of such approaches at present are given below.

The second stage at which immunological control may be exerted is after the establishment of a primary tumour. At this stage the host may exert some control over the spread of the tumour, especially by limiting metastases. The phenomenon of concomitant immunity in experimental animals provides a model in which such control can be studied. The treatment of tumours solely by immunological means at this stage would constitute true immunotherapy and although this seems feasible with some experimental tumours few, if any, immunologists would advocate its use in man.

The third stage for control is after treatment of the disease by other means. It is logical to use immunotherapy as an adjunct to conventional treatment, when the residual tumour burden has been reduced as far as possible by that treatment (Woodruff, 1970). Immunotherapy is, however, sometimes used as a last resort in patients with disseminated disease uncontrolled by other means. Two approaches are possible, either singly or together: specific immunotherapy, in which attempts are made to boost immunity towards tumour cells; and non-specific immunotherapy, in which attempts are made to boost immune responsiveness in general. A rational approach to immunoprophylaxis, immunopotentiation and immunotherapy requires some consideration of the mechanisms of immunological resistance to cancer and of the immunological status of the tumour-bearing host.

Mechanisms of immunological resistance to cancer

It is unusual for an antigen to excite a single 'immune response'. Commonly, a range of diverse immune responses occurs. The range may include the production of antibodies of different functional types, the development of cell-mediated immunity involving specifically reactive effector lymphocytes, which may be functionally heterogeneous, and combined humoral and cell-mediated responses. Tumour cells – in man and experimental animals – can induce a full range of immune responses. The mechanisms available to the host are thus also diverse. Effective expression of immunological resistance to cancer may require the harmonious combination of several responses. Conversely, potent effector mechanisms may be rendered inoperative or 'blocked' in various ways, especially by antibodies which do not themselves trigger an attack on target tumour cells.

The mechanisms of expression of immunity to tumours have been discussed in several recent reviews (Cerottini and Brunner, 1974; Hellström and Hellström, 1974; Nelson, 1974; Evans and Alexander, 1976). They have been elucidated by a combination of approaches involving cell separation and testing of anti-tumour activity in vivo and in vitro, notably by assays of cytotoxicity using ^{51}Cr release from labelled target cells or target cell survival in microculture. They include:

1. Direct and specific cytotoxicity effected by T cells alone.

2. A cytotoxic effect specifically initiated by T cells but requiring the participation of macrophages as helper cells.

3. A non-specific cytotoxic effect exerted on tumour cells of any kind, but not on normal cells, by activated macrophages ('activation' implies increases in antimicrobial activity, metabolic activity generally, size and the content of intracellular organelles).

4. A cytotoxic effect initiated by antibodies directed specifically at antigens on the tumour cell surface, but ultimately effected by complement, by macrophages, or by a specialised sub-class of lymphoid cells called 'K' ('killer') cells; in the last case the antibody is referred to as lymphocyte-dependent antibody.

5. A direct and specific cytotoxic effect of B cells; it is still unclear whether this is a real mechanism, or an apparent one involving B cells synthesising lymphocyte-dependent antibody which then collaborates with K cells.

There is abundant information about the nature and mode of action of cytotoxic T cells. They are extremely potent effector cells in allogeneic systems. There is a surprising paucity of information about their roles in resistance to syngeneic or autochthonous tumours. There is, indeed, a suspicion that 'successful' tumours are relatively resistant to direct T cell attack, amplification by macrophages being required (Kearney et al., 1975; Simes et al., 1975).

The concept of blocking of the expression of tumour immunity is central to current thinking on the subject. Mechanisms of blocking include: the presence of excess tumour antigen in soluble form masking receptors on specifically reactive cells or antibodies; the presence of antibodies which themselves cannot initiate attack on tumour cells but which cover antigens on the tumour cells so that they are not 'seen' by other antibodies or by effector lymphocytes; and the presence of complexes of soluble tumour antigens and antibodies. The last of these three seems more potent than the others.

From the existence of diverse effector mechanisms and of blocking factors it follows that rational immunological control of a tumour is aimed at stimulating a mechanism most likely to bring about destruction of tumour cells, without stimulating the formation of blocking antibodies.

Immunological status of the tumour-bearing host

Experimental animals bearing tumours of autochthonous or (more commonly) syngeneic origin may possess lymphoid cells capable of reacting with and destroying the cells of the tumour in culture. In some cases, e.g. with some Moloney virus-induced tumours in mice, this reactivity may be adequate to bring about regression of the tumour. In others, e.g. many chemically induced fibrosarcomas in mice, reactivity may be inadequate or may be blocked (Hellström and Hellström, 1974; Lamon et al., 1974). The general immunological status of tumour-bearing animals may also be changed. Mice bearing chemically or virally induced tumours may show depressed primary antibody production and depressed cell-mediated immunity (Wells et al., 1974; Kirchner et al., 1975). The lymphoid cell balance may be grossly disturbed with increases, relative or absolute, in the numbers of B cells and macrophages and a decrease in the number of T cells (Smith and Konda, 1973; Kirchner et al., 1975).

As with mice, so with men. Patients with cancer may possess circulating lymphoid cells capable of destroying target tumour cells in vitro and they may also possess blocking antibodies. There is, furthermore, suggestive evidence that the outcome for the host may be reflected in or determined by the balance between the two (Hellström and Hellström, 1974; Heppner, 1973; Herberman, 1974), although the validity of some of the commonly used techniques has been called in question (Takasugi et al., 1973). Immunological reactivity may be non-specifically affected, with depression of antibody production and cell-mediated immunity (Hersh et al., 1974; Eilber et al., 1975; Lee et al., 1975), a decrease in the number of circulating T cells (Anthony et al., 1975) and an increase in macrophage numbers or activity (Magarey and Baum, 1970).

Thus, attempts at immunotherapy are of necessity carried out in patients whose immune systems are already altered in two ways: they may already have made a primary response, humoral and/or cell-mediated, to tumour specific antigens; and they may have significant impairment of their capacity to respond.

Immunoprophylaxis

Certain viruses can cause cancer in experimental animals, notably in laboratory rodents. Resistance to the oncogenic effects of some of these viruses may be induced by specific immunization. There is an abundance of evidence consistent with the notion that viruses are causative agents of some human malignant diseases: type C RNA viruses in acute leukaemia (Harris, 1973; Gallo et al., 1974); a type B virus in carcinoma of the breast (Moore, 1974; Henderson, 1974); Epstein-Barr virus, a herpesvirus, in Burkitt's lymphoma (Henle and Henle, 1974; Rapp, 1974); and herpesvirus type 2 (herpes simplex virus type 2) in carcinoma of the uterine cervix (Melnick et al., 1974; Rapp, 1974). The gap between work in laboratory rodents and practical preventive medicine for man has been narrowed somewhat by the recent report of successful vaccination of cotton-topped marmosets against a malignant lymphoma by means of a killed vaccine of the causative agent, herpesvirus saimiri (Laufs and Steinke, 1975). Nevertheless there are serious theoretical and practical difficulties in the way of human cancer control by means of virus vaccines, even if a particular virus were shown to cause a particular form of cancer. Laboratory manipulation may have created defective particles, whose number may have been increased by inactivation and which could, on inoculation by an unnatural route, cause malignant transformation (Rapp and Buss, 1974). If a vertically transmitted virus caused a human malignancy, e.g. acute leukaemia or breast cancer, the putatively normal cells might carry virus or viral antigens for some years before the emergence of frank malignancy. Active immunization might in such circumstances be followed by a vigorous attack on the normal cells, with disastrous consequences. When only a small proportion of virus-infected persons develop tumours, the costs of developing and producing a vaccine and of either identifying a high-risk group or vaccinating a very large population may be prohibitive. The development of specific immunoprophylactic measures against forms of cancer not induced by viruses, e.g. chemically induced tumours, is open to the same practical objections. It is also open to the theoretical objection that the major strong antigens of chemically induced tumours are individual-specific, the common antigens being less immunogenic (Baldwin, 1973; Kearney and Nelson, 1973).

Another approach to immunoprophylaxis involves the concept of immunological surveillance. This is the concept that the immune system is constantly operating to recognise and react against antigenically altered, potentially malignant mutant cells (Burnet, 1970). The surveillance might be exercised by T cells, as commonly supposed, or by macrophages, especially those in an activated state. The best evidence that surveillance exists is the increased occurrence of malignant disease in immunosuppressed renal transplant recipients and in patients with immunodeficiency (Penn, 1970; Good, 1971). Many of these tumours are lymphoid and it may be argued that chronic antigenic stimulation plays a part in their genesis. A significant number are, however, of epithelial origin. Skin tumours, for example, are important causes of morbidity in Australian transplant recipients (Australian National Renal Transplantation Survey, 1974). On the other hand, it has been argued that surveillance is unimportant, partly because of the unchanged incidence of spontaneous tumours in nude mice which lack T cells (Prehn, 1974). In such mice, however, macrophages may be sufficiently stimulated to exercise surveillance. It is possible in experimental animals to increase resistance to syngeneic tumours by means of agents with an immunopotentiating effect (Yashphe, 1972). Such agents as BCG vaccine are now included in experimental immunotherapeutic regimes in man (see below). One series of observations suggested that BCG vaccination increased the resistance of children in Canada to leukaemogenesis (Davignon et al., 1970), but this has not been found to hold good elsewhere.

Immunological resistance to the spread of cancer: concomitant immunity

Distant metastases may be suppressed even in patients in whose circulation tumour cells have been found. The limitation or suppression of secondary tumours can be studied in experimental animals which exhibit concomitant immunity. This term refers to the ability of animals bearing a tumour isograft to reject a second graft from the same tumour. The phenomenon has been observed with a variety of tumours in mice, hamsters and rats (Nelson, 1974). In many cases, notably with lymphomas in hamsters and methylcholanthrene-induced tumours in mice, resistance to a second induced tumour graft is greater while the primary isograft is in place than after its surgical removal. In mice concomitant immunity is thymus-dependent and cell-mediated. In thymus-deprived animals concomitant immunity did not occur and normally non-metastasizing tumours gave rise to metastases. Conversely, tumours which did not induce concomitant immunity tended to metastasize (Kearney and Nelson, 1973; Kearney et al., 1975). The existence of this phenomenon provides very clear experimental evidence for the existence of immunological mechanisms controlling tumour spread as opposed to tumour emergence.

Immunotherapy and immunopotentiation

Immunotherapy of human malignant disease is generally an adjunct to conventional treatment by means of surgery, radiotherapy and/or chemotherapy. The term immunotherapy is often applied somewhat loosely to those studies in experimental animals in which animals receive treatment before challenge with tumour cells. Such studies are useful in providing models in which potentially useful agents can be tested. Immunopotentiation is, however, a more useful term to embrace studies in model systems and in man. It would be impossible even to survey here the wide range of approaches to immunopotentiation and immunotherapy. Instead, a summary of some principles and some key findings will be given (for reviews, see Yashphe, 1972; Baker and Taub, 1973; Currie, 1974; Mathé and Weiner, 1974; Bast et al., *Lancet,* 1974, 1975; McKhann and Gunnarson, 1974).

A wide variety of agents injected into experimental animals before or, in some cases, with or just after challenge with a tumour can induce partial or complete resistance to the challenge. These include BCG vaccine and other mycobacteria or mycobacterial extracts, other microbes such as *Corynebacterium parvum,* interferon and natural or synthetic products such as pyran, lentinan and levamisole. Many, if not all, of these agents act as immunological adjuvants and stimulate cells of the mononuclear phagocytic system. It is usually not possible to decide whether the agents act as adjuvants promoting a specific response to the tumour antigens, as sources of antigen cross-reacting with tumour antigens, or as inducers of activated macrophages which then kill tumour cells in a relatively non-specific fashion. These possibilities are not mutually exclusive. In one model system – BCG and a mastocytoma in mice – the induction of resistance required the injection of both BCG and tumour cells, suggesting a requirement for specific antigen as well as adjuvant or stimulant of the mononuclear phagocytic system (Hawrylko and Mackaness, 1973a,b).

An immunopotentiating agent effective against one tumour may not be effective against another. Levamisole treatment had a marked effect on the Lewis lung tumour in mice (Renoux and Renoux, 1972) but had no effect on two virus-induced tumours of mice, a virus-induced tumour of hamsters or a chemically induced tumour of rats (Potter et al., 1974). It induced resistance to only one of six methylcholanthrene-induced fibrosarcomas in mice (D.S. Nelson and J. M. Penrose, unpublished results).

Immunopotentiating agents may be effective in hosts lacking full immunological competence. This has been found with *C. parvum* in T cell-deprived mice (Woodruff et al., 1973), pyran co-polymer in mice treated with anti-lymphocyte serum (Hirsch et al., 1973) and with BCG in cyclophosphamide-treated mice

(Houchens et al., 1974) and athymic nude mice (Pimm and Baldwin, 1975). While these findings raise questions about the mode of action of the agents examined, they also provide an encouraging background for immunopotentiation in human patients, whose immune responsiveness is frequently depressed.

Inappropriate timing of the administration of immunopotentiating agents may have the paradoxical effect of reducing resistance and facilitating tumour growth. This has been observed with BCG and mammary tumours in rats (Piessens et al., 1970).

Specific immunopotentiation or immunotherapy has been achieved by the injection of tumour cells treated with neuraminidase in mice (Simmons and Rios, 1974) and dogs (Sedlacek et al., 1975). This approach probably deserves more attention than it has received in human studies.

Trials of immunotherapy in several human malignant diseases have been undertaken. The most extensive have involved the use of BCG, with or without irradiated tumour cells. The results with patients with acute leukaemia have been good in that patients who entered remission after reductive chemotherapy remained in remission longer with immunotherapy than without (Mathé et al., 1969, 1974; Powles et al., 1973). Encouraging results have also been obtained with patients with disseminated melanoma, although such patients, bearing a large tumour load, are not ideal candidates for immunotherapy (Mavligit et al., 1974). Limited trials with other tumours have given results which, while not clearcut, range from the inconclusive to the encouraging (Baker and Taub, 1973). It is well known that other trials of BCG with or without irradiated or otherwise modified tumour cells are under way, but the natural history of cancer is such that valid results cannot be expected for some time.

Other approaches are also being made to immunotherapy and immunopotentiation in man. Transfer factor prepared from lymphocytes confers upon the recipients the cell-mediated immune reactivity of the donor. Its use has given encouraging results in osteogenic sarcoma (Levin et al., 1975), though the results with other tumours are difficult to assess because of the small numbers of patients or the lack of adequate controls (Basten et al., 1975). Levamisole has been found to increase cell-mediated immune responsiveness of patients with advanced cancer (Tripodi et al., 1973; P. Hersey, G. W. Milton and D. S. Nelson, unpublished results). This effect, plus its apparent safety, justifies more extended trials. More attention is also being paid to the possibility of removing blocking antibody by plasmaphoresis and selectively suppressing the synthesis of more blocking antibody by means of drugs such as cyclophosphamide. In theory this should allow existing effector lymphocytes to attack the tumour cells without hindrance.

The ethics of experimental therapeutics and the difficulties of conducting controlled trials are subjects of perennial concern to all charged with the care of patients with life-threatening diseases (Chalmers et al., 1972; Strauss, 1973). It seems ethically mandatory that trials of any form of immunological intervention in cancer should be adequately controlled, in the statistical sense, so that the results are meaningful, and adequately monitored by laboratory tests so that parameters of good, or bad, responses can be identified.

References

Anthony, H. M., Kirk, J. A., Madsen, E., Mason, M. K. and Templeman, G. H. (1975): *Clin. exp. Immunol., 20,* 29.

Australian National Renal Transplantation Survey (1974): *Med. J. Aust., 2,* 656.

Baker, M. A. and Taub, R. N. (1973): *Progr. Allergy, 17,* 227.

Baldwin, R. W. (1973): *Advanc. Cancer Res., 18,* 1.

Bast, R. C., Zbar, B., Borsos, T. and Rapp, H. J. (1974): *New Engl. J. Med., 290,* 1413 and 1458.

Basten, A., Croft, S., Kenny, D. F. and Nelson, D. S. (1975): *Vox Sang. (Basel), 28,* 257.

Burnet, F. M. (1970): *Immunological Surveillance.* Pergamon Press, Sydney.

Cerottini, J.-C. and Brunner, K. T. (1974): *Advanc. Immunol., 18,* 67.

Chalmers, T. C., Block, J. B. and Lee, S. (1972): *New Engl. J. Med., 287,* 75.

Currie, G. A. (1974): *Cancer and the Immune Response,* Chapter 7, p. 71. Edward Arnold, London.

Davignon, L., Lemonde, P., Robillard, P. and Frappier, A. (1971): *Lancet, 1,* 80.

Eilber, F. R., Nizze, J. A. and Morton, D. L. (1975): *Cancer (Philad.), 35,* 660.

Evans, R. and Alexander, P. (1976): In: *Immunobiology of the Macrophage,* p. 536. Editor: D. S. Nelson. Academic Press, New York.

Gallo, R. C., Gallagher, R. E., Sarngadharan, M. G., Sarin, P., Reitz, M., Miller, N. and Gillespie, D. H. (1974): *Cancer (Philad.), 34,* 1398.

Good, R. A. (1971): *Harvey Lect., 67,* 1.

Harris, R. (1973): *Nature (Lond.), 241,* 95.

Hawrylko, E. and Mackaness, G. B. (1973a): *J. nat. Cancer Inst., 51,* 1677.

Hawrylko, E. and Mackaness, G. B. (1973b): *J. nat. Cancer Inst., 51,* 1683.

Hellström, K. E. and Hellström, I. (1974): *Advanc. Immunol., 18,* 209.

Henderson, B. E. (1974): *Cancer (Philad.), 34,* 1386.

Henle, W. and Henle, G. (1974): *Cancer (Philad.), 34,* 1368.

Heppner, G. H. (1973): In: *Breast Cancer: A Challenging Problem,* p. 63. Editors: M. L. Griem, E. V. Jensen, J. E. Ultmann and R. W. Wissler. Springer-Verlag, Berlin.

Herberman, R. B. (1974): *Advanc. Cancer Res., 19,* 207.

Hersh, E. M., Freireich, E. J., McCredie, K. B., Gutterman, J. V., Bodey, G. P., White-car, J. P., Mavligit, G. and Cheema, A. R. (1974): In: *Investigation and Stimulation of Immunity in Cancer Patients,* p. 25. Editors: G. Mathé and R. Weiner. Springer-Verlag, Berlin.

Hirsch, M. S., Black, P. H., Wood, M. L. and Monaco, A. P. (1973): *J. Immunol., 111,* 91.

Houchens, D. P., Gaston, M. R., Kinney, Y. and Goldin, A. (1974): *Cancer Chemother. Rep., 58,* 931.

Kearney, R., Basten, A. and Nelson, D. S. (1975): *Int. J. Cancer, 15,* 438.

Kearney, R. and Nelson, D. S. (1973). *Aust. J. exp. Biol. med. Sci., 51,* 723.

Kirchner, H., Muchmore, A. V., Chused, T. M., Holden, H. T. and Herberman, R. B. (1975): *J. Immunol., 114,* 206.

Lamon, E. W., Andersson, B., Wigzell, H., Fenyö, E. M. and Klein, E. (1974): *Int. J. Cancer, 13,* 91.

Lancet (1974): Leading article, *1,* 846.

Lancet (1975): Leading article, *1,* 151.

Laufs, R. and Steinke, H. (1975): *Nature (Lond.), 253,* 71.

Lee, Y. T., Sparks, F. C., Eilber, F. R. and Morton, D. L. (1975): *Cancer (Philad.), 35,* 748.

Levin, A. S., Byers, V. S., Fudenberg, H. H., Wybran, J., Hackett, A. J., Johnston, J. O. and Spitler, L. E. (1975): *J. clin. Invest., 55,* 487.

Lindenmann, J. (1974): *Biochim. biophys. Acta Rev. Cancer, 355,* 49.

McKhann, C. F. and Gunnarson, A. (1974): *Cancer (Philad.), 34,* 1521.

Magarey, C. J. and Baum, M. (1970): *Brit. J. Surg., 57,* 748.

Mathé, G., Amiel, J. L., Schwarzenberg, L., Schneider, M., Cattan, A., Schlumberger, J. R., Hayat, M. and de Vassal, F. (1969): *Lancet, 1,* 697.

Mathé, G., Pouillart, P., Schwarzenberg, L., Weiner, R., Rappaport, H., Hayat, M., de Vassal, F., Amiel, J. L., Schneider, M., Jasmin, C. and Rosenfeld, C. (1974): In: *Investigation and Stimulation of Immunity in Cancer Patients,* p. 434. Editors: G. Mathé and R. Weiner. Springer-Verlag, Berlin.

Mathé, G. and Weiner, R. (Ed.) (1974): *Investigation and Stimulation of Immunity in Cancer Patients.* Springer-Verlag, Berlin.

Mavligit, G., Gutterman, J. V., McBride, C. and Hersh, E. M. (1974): *Progr. exp. Tumor Res., 19,* 222.

Melnick, J. L., Adam, E. and Rawls, W. E. (1974): *Cancer (Philad.), 34,* 1375.

Moore, D. H. (1974): *Cancer Res., 34,* 2322.

Nelson, D. S. (1974): *Transplant. Rev., 19,* 226.

Penn, I. (1970): *Malignant Tumors in Organ Transplant Recipients.* Springer-Verlag, Berlin.

Piessens, W. F., Lachapelle, F. L., Legros, N. and Heuson, J. C. (1970): *Nature (Lond.), 228,* 1210.

Pimm, M. V. and Baldwin, R. W. (1975): *Nature (Lond.), 254,* 77.

Potter, C. W., Carr, I., Jennings, R., Rees, R. C., McGinty, F. and Richardson, V. M. (1974): *Nature (Lond.), 249,* 567.

Powles, R. L., Crowther, D., Bateman, C. J. T., Beard, M. E. J., McElwain, T. J., Russel, J., Lister, T. A., Whitehouse, J. M. A., Wrigley, P. F. M., Pike, M. C., Alexander, P. and Fairley, G. H. (1973): *Brit. J. Cancer, 28,* 365.

Prehn, R. T. (1974): *Amer. J. Path., 77,* 119.

Rapp, F. (1974): *Advanc. Cancer Res., 19,* 265.

Rapp, F. and Buss, E. R. (1974): *Amer. J. Path., 77,* 85.

Renoux, G. and Renoux, M. (1972): *Nature new Biol., 240,* 217.

Roberts, S. S., Hengesh, J. W., McGrath, R. G., Valaitis, J., McGrew, E. A. and Cole, W. H. (1967): *Amer. J. Surg., 113,* 757.

Sedlacek, H. H., Meesmann, H. and Seiler, F. R. (1975): *Int. J. Cancer, 15,* 409.

Simes, R. J., Kearney, R. and Nelson, D. S. (1975): *Immunology, 29,* 343.

Simmons, R. L. and Rios, A. (1974): *Cancer (Philad.), 34,* 1541.

Smith, R. T. (1972): *New Engl. J. Med., 287,* 439.

Smith, R. T. and Konda, S. (1973): *Int. J. Cancer, 12,* 577.

Strauss, M. B. (1973): *New Engl. J. Med., 288,* 1183.

Takasugi, M., Mickey, M. R. and Terasaki, P. (1973): *Cancer Res., 33,* 2898.

Tripodi, D., Parks, L. C. and Brugmans, J. (1973): *New Engl. J. Med., 289,* 354.

Wells, J. H., Cain, W. A., Wells, R. S. and Bozalis, J. R. (1974): *Int. Arch. Allergy, 47,* 362.

Woodruff, M. (1970): *Harvey Lect., 66,* 161.

Woodruff, M., Dunbar, N. and Ghaffar, A. (1973): *Proc. roy. Soc. B, 184,* 97.

Yashphe, D. J. (1972): In: *Immunological Parameters of Host-Tumor Relationships,* p. 90. Editor: D. W. Weiss. Academic Press, New York.

7: The clinical laboratory 1975-1984

Quality control: the next five years

B. E. Copeland

Laboratory of Pathology, New England Deaconess Hospital, Boston, Mass.,
U.S.A.

In the next five years quality control will continue to develop and expand to include all laboratories doing tests for patient care. This will include the physician's office doing screening tests as well as the research laboratory which does an occasional unusual test for patient care.

Universal acceptance of day-to-day quality control

Day-to-day quality control of each test will become universally accepted. This will apply not only in chemistry, but in every other discipline of the laboratory. This will extend from such simple tests as the occult blood test in the stool to such complex tests as the serum ACTH or the identification of carcinoma in a histologic tissue section.

Some new areas of quality control will develop such as quality control of the educational process. How effective is our education? One example from my own experience shows that in a parasitology textbook only one sentence in forty was of diagnostic importance.

There will be an extension of quality control to include: (1) the selection of the test, (2) collection and processing of samples prior to testing, (3) the entire reporting system, (4) and finally the quality control of the use of the test in patient management. This will require ingenuity and creative development.

It would be encouraging to see quality control concepts taught thoroughly in schools of medical technology, as well as in medical school. It would be beneficial to include quality control concepts in science courses in grammar school and secondary schools. In the area of chemistry we will see extension of large regional quality control programmes. In the United States the regional control programmes are now widely developed, so that a majority of hospital laboratories are now participating in these programmes. The two major advantages are: (1) cost-purchase of 300 litre pools is much less expensive than 3 litre amounts; (2) monthly comparison of results among 50-250 hospital laboratories allows a decision to be made as to the interchangeability of results between hospitals.

Quality control will extend to include instrument maintenance programmes in order to improve performance by effective preventive action.

Quality control will become more patient orientated – as federal regulation and accreditation programmes increase it will be necessary to focus on the patient benefit derived from the regulations. In my experience in two instances in the past five years two specific regulations by the Federal Government and the College of American Pathologists (CAP) have been shown to be unnecessary. The first was a requirement for concomitant gram-positive and -negative controls with each gram stain; no laboratory followed this requirement and it was dropped. A similar requirement of the CAP that 10% of normal vaginal pap smears must be reinspected by a pathologist was felt by many to be an inappropriate use of resources. It is now being revised.

These are examples of cost-benefit evaluation of specific regulations. The system works best when there is a dynamic relationship between the regulator and those regulated.

Quality control will assist in maintaining the medical heritage which relates the disease entity to the diagnostic test by eliminating bias from methods and instruments. For example, the diagnosis of the parathyroid tumour was associated with serum calcium levels after the tumour was discovered. The continued use of serum calcium depends on its continued effectiveness in predicting parathyroid tumours. Quality control of any bias introduced by new methods or instruments is important.

Quality control at the editorial level is also necessary. New methods and instruments require evaluation for bias in relation to reference methods. In this regard editorial quality control is a necessary new development.

The limitations of external quality control will be recognized. As pointed out by Eldjarn of Norway, after four years of an external control programme the improvement curve levels off at between 80 and 90%. Subsequent progress in quality control of the external quality control samples themselves will become a recognized necessity. This is due to the problem of preparing test materials which are homogeneous, and which maintain specific diagnostic characteristics.

Quality control of manufactured products will be recognized as a highly important activity. Such improvement in the reliability of manufactured products will show direct benefit in the laboratory performance. Concomitant with the quality control of manufactured products will be quality control of the delivery of these products to the user. Replacement parts and repair services are needed immediately for good patient care.

The standards for export of reagents and instruments adopted by the Commission on World Standards of the World Association of Societies of Pathology will serve as a quality control in this area. Each country should adopt a rule of strict quality control policy in this area.

In conclusion, during the next five years quality control in the clinical laboratory will expand to include the manufacturers and distributors of laboratory products, the practising physician who does simple laboratory tests, as well as all aspects of the pathology laboratory itself.

Medical usefulness of laboratory testing

R. N. Barnett

Norwalk Hospital, Norwalk, Conn., U.S.A.

I would like to use the relatively brief time at my disposal to outline some of the important aspects of this subject. I will comment on the status of some of the studies of the Council on Quality Assurance of the College of American Pathologists, encompassing a number of Commissions and Committees, most of whose activities are directly pertinent to the subject of medical usefulness.

How tests are used: sensitivity, specificity and interpretation

This covers a variety of disciplines but we are interested in the unifying approach which the pathologist brings. Individual clinicians may use tests very well in making specific decisions; however their approach is frequently entirely pragmatic and nonphilosophical. Pathologists should know in considerable detail the accuracy and precision of their own tests, their proneness to blatant errors and their performance in many diagnostic situations. Interpretation is much more meaningful when we have these tools.

Screening tests

Our Medical Usefulness Subcommittee has considered this subject and pointed out some of the problems (Barnett et al., 1970). This information needs updating. We should now be in a position to consider new screening tests and groups of tests and to retire the less useful ones instead of merely buying bigger machines to spew forth more results. We need to develop cost-effectiveness studies as to how screening batteries work in different clinical situations. The finding that the recommended sixth test for occult blood in the stool costs 47 million dollars to find a new case of colon cancer speaks for itself! (Neuhauser and Sewicki, 1975).

Communication of results to the clinician

Our Subcommittee published a brief and rather general set of guidelines for this subject, covering chiefly what a report should be (Burns et al., 1974). We did not cover such aspects as the frequently slow pace of reporting (Barnett et al., 1975). Computerization of reports makes possible many new arrangements of data; we need to contemplate these before the field becomes static.

Patient preparation, specimen collection and handling

Again our group has addressed this problem and the College of American Pathologists has two publications available. One merely covers venipuncture (*So You're Going to Collect a Blood Specimen,* 1974); the other discusses the more general factors (Schoen et al., 1974). Probably more poor test results occur because of inept handling of specimens than because of inadequate analyses, and we require continuing monitoring in this field. We certainly can't memorize Dr. Young's 17,000 chemical interferences (Young et al., 1975), but we can discourage drawing samples under suboptimal conditions.

Nomenclature

The College of American Pathologists has produced a Systematized Nomenclature of Pathology (SNOP) which is widely used for coding medical diagnoses. It is presently being expanded with SNOMed, a version which includes diagnostic tests and treatments. The first field test of this will take place early next year. I am avoiding the subject of SI units as being too controversial for discussion here.

'Normal' values

Physicians must have some frame of reference against which to measure test results, whatever name we give this frame. The Standards Commission is proceeding with a conference early this Winter at which we will attempt to plan strategy for some practical approach to the problem, in the full knowledge that many others have tried this approach and failed.

Documentation that laboratory data have been observed and evaluated

Our Committee, chaired by Dr. Sara Winter, has been rewording a statement with this title for over a year. It has now been submitted to *Pathologist,* The College of American Pathologists' magazine, for publication. The subject has important medical and legal ramifications; test results not delivered or noted are not very helpful!

Use of blood transfusions

Although transfusion therapy itself is a subject requiring input from many types of medical specialties, there are certain specific areas which pathologists should be investigating. These include at least the types of blood products, the laboratory monitoring of responses, and the decisions about giving blood when the crossmatching is incompatible to some degree.

Elimination of poor tests in favor of better ones

All too often a new better test is merely added on to the obsolete test. Only rarely have clear-cut recommendations been made to just stop doing poor tests (Kim and Barnett, 1974). We all know that flame photometry for calcium is very inaccurate, but not enough of us have said so. At a certain point our societies should take a definite stand in this area.

How physicians use tests

We are presently studying a specific aspect of this, namely the degree of change which clinicians believe to be significant. We posed a series of specific clinical problems and asked whether a fall of, for example, 2 or 4 or 6 mg would lead them to take positive action. After a preliminary random sample of 125 internists we are now querying a group of 500 general practioners.

Guidelines for appropriate utilization of tests

We have a College of American Pathologists Committee specifically to study this subject. Although it was originally established to deal with Professional Review Organizations, it is rapidly spreading out into choice of tests, frequency of repetition and field studies of the values found in specific clinical situations.

As you can see there is no lack of subjects. Although I have used the frame of reference of clinical chemistry and hematology primarily, there are similar problems in cytology, microbiology and all our other fields. We welcome any ideas you wish to bring to the Subcommittee on Medical Usefulness of COWS-WASP and any volunteers to undertake specific studies.

References

Barnett, R. N., Bimmell, M., Peracca, M. and Rosemann, K. (1975): *Pathologist, 3-8,* January.
Barnett, R. N., Civin, W. H. and Schoen, I. (1970): *Amer. J. clin. Path., 54,* 483.
Burns, E. L., Hanson, D. J., Schoen, I., Minckler, T. and Winter, S. (1974): *Amer. J. clin. Path., 61,* 900.
Kim, H. and Barnett, R. N. (1974): *Amer. J. clin. Path., 61,* 139.
Neuhauser, D. and Sewicki, A. M. (1975): *New Engl. J. Med., 293,* 226.
Schoen, I., Fischer, C., Winter, S. and Barnett, R. N. (1974): *Documentation that Laboratory Results Have Been Delivered and Noted.* College of American Pathologists.
Young, D. M., Pestaner, L. C. and Gibberman, V. (1975): *Clin. Chem., 21,* 1D.

Thoughts on cost effectiveness in laboratory testing

D. B. Dorsey

Department of Pathology, Central du Page Hospital, Winfield, Ill., U.S.A.

If we are to discuss the concept of cost effectiveness in laboratory testing in any meaningful way, we must evaluate all the elements of cost associated with the testing process and consider the cost and value of what happens as a result of that testing. The costs directly associated with testing a specimen, listed in Table 1, include only expenses incurred in the laboratory and may actually represent a small component of total costs. Associated costs, shown in Table 2, are an indispensable part of the testing process. The total of these associated costs may exceed the cost of running the test.

When testing is done in a hospital, the patient benefits directly or indirectly

TABLE 1

Laboratory costs

1. Instrument purchase or lease	6. Direction and supervision
2. Instrument maintenance	7. Payroll and fringes
3. Reagents and standards	8. Professional compensation
4. Supplies	9. Overhead
5. Quality control programs	10. Return on investment

from many services paid for partially or wholly by laboratory fees. These service costs, shown in Table 3, are part of the legitimate expenses of laboratory testing.

In addition to costs concerned with the testing process, other costs must be considered. These expenses, shown in Table 4, are related to what happens as a result of testing.

TABLE 2

Associated costs

1. Producing and transmitting the requisition
2. Obtaining, processing and transporting the specimen
3. Evaluating, interpreting, transmitting and filing the report
4. Data processing
5. Billing and collecting fees
6. Bad debts

TABLE 3

Service costs

1. Pathologist's consultations – formal and informal
2. The 'free' autopsy service
3. Technical and professional support of essential hospital and medical quality control programs:

Infection Surveillance	Audit Committee
Tumor Boards	Transfusion Committee
Death Conferences	Bed Utilization Committee
Clinical Pathological Conferences	Tissue Committee

4. Educational programs for:

Clinicians	Nurses
House Staff	Other Paramedics
Technical Staff	Etc.

TABLE 4

Related costs

1. Re-testing of equivocal results
2. Follow-up testing of positives
3. Related diagnostic procedures
4. Physician's examinations and consultations
5. Medical and surgical therapy
6. Therapeutic monitoring
7. Therapeutic follow-up and re-testing

TABLE 5

Objectives of testing in the Public Health setting

1. To identify and define environmental risk factors (infectious agents, toxic chemicals, etc.)
2. To evaluate and monitor susceptibility of populations at risk
3. To evaluate the association between elements of heredity and lifestyle, such as race, nutrition, tobacco and alcohol and the occurrence of disease

In addition to including all elements of cost, we must define 'effectiveness'. Effectiveness is determined by how well we achieve the goals and objectives of testing. Since we are concerned with laboratory testing related to health, our goals must be health-related. Health testing is done in four distinct settings, each with clearly defined objectives. As objectives vary, so determinants of cost effectiveness of laboratory testing vary with the setting.

Laboratory testing in the public health setting

The objectives of testing in the public health setting are listed in Table 5. Mechanic (1975) states: 'Every person who works in the area of social medicine realizes that medical care, as more narrowly defined, has only a peripheral effect on health in populations – increases in longevity and reductions in mortality depend to a major extent on improvements in the quality of the environment'.

Laboratory testing in the public health setting to identify environmental risks, extrapolates test results to hundreds, thousands or millions of persons at risk with tremendous leverage for good. If cost effectiveness is evaluated in terms of the number of lives improved or prolonged per test performed or per dollar spent, this segment of laboratory testing must be judged by far the most 'cost effective'.

Peery (1975), in his Ward Burdick address, illustrated the dramatic decrease in infectious disease mortality achieved by public health measures before antibiotics were developed. Figure 1 from his presentation illustrates this graphically. The arrow indicates the beginning of the antibiotic era.

Testing to evaluate the association between elements of lifestyle and the occurrence of disease is likely to be much less cost effective – partly because much more extensive testing is required to establish the association with reasonable certainty, and partly because knowledge of the correlation has little effect on behavior – witness the increasing use of cigarettes and the rising incidence of

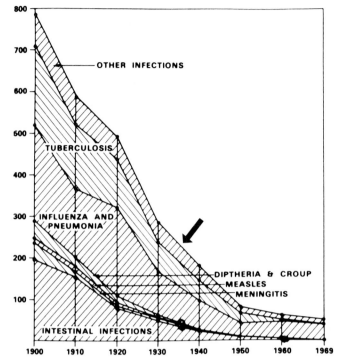

Fig. 1. U.S.A. death rates for infections 1900-1969. From Peery (1975); courtesy of the editors *Amer. J. clin. Path.*

smoking-related illness in the U.S.A. in spite of 11 years of health hazard warnings printed on every pack!

Laboratory testing in a health screening setting

The objective of testing in the health screening setting is to assess personal health risks and identify anatomic and physiologic deviations, including metabolic defects, likely to be harbingers of disease in symptomless individuals.

The 'cost effectiveness' of laboratory testing in the screening mode has been more extensively studied than any other, and yet conclusions are still ambiguous and controversial. Problems concern both comprehensive cost analysis and the clear definition and comparative evaluation of benefits (effectiveness).

Collen et al. (1970) have determined the dollar cost per positive test in a comprehensive screening program. This simplistic approach neither includes all related costs nor evaluates the effectiveness of a positive test finding. Paulus et al. (1970) point out that abnormal data generated by a routine laboratory screening program do not confirm a diagnosis or justify therapy, but merely represent a different type of 'chief complaint' which must be carefully investigated before a diagnosis is made or therapy started.

The cost and effectiveness of testing for a disease must include the cost of confirmation, follow-up and therapy, because, as Wolf (1972) points out, 'there is little purpose in discovering disease unless one is prepared to take appropriate action'. In fact, unless specific means of prevention or treatment are available, the cost of testing seems unjustifiable; if treatment is available, the cost of therapy and follow-up must be considered as part of the comprehensive cost.

How can we quantitate the benefits (and cost effectiveness) of health screening? Emlet (1968) proposed 'extended years of chronic disease-free, or disease-controlled life per dollar' and 'the total gain in federal income tax revenues due to extended life and reduced disability'. Bush (1972) suggests savings on the cost of institutionalization resulting from early treatment (of infants with phenylketonuria). Collen et al. (1973) use lower disability and mortality rates for a defined population group (middle-aged men).

An AMA statement on multiphasic health testing proposes other, less quantifiable benefits, such as improved medical records, better use of physician's time, earlier detection of asymptomatic disease, service to more patients, improved data base, and improved health education.

The yield of the screening process is influenced by the specificity and sensitivity of the test and by disease incidence. Werner et al. (1973) point out that a multiphasic screening problem concerns the fact that diagnostic sensitivity decreases with decreasing incidence of the sought disease, so that the few true positives are diluted with relatively large numbers of false positives.

On the other hand, when disease incidence is low, the few false negatives have a negligible effect on the large number of true negatives. These 'dilution' effects increase the specificity of the test and favor the 'ruling out', but not the 'ruling in', of a condition. Very few true positives will be missed, but when large 'healthy' populations undergo multiphasic screening, the economic consequences of follow-up on numerous 'false positives' may be intolerable.

A critical determinant in the value and cost effectiveness of health screening concerns the cost of what will happen if the disease is not detected. This is illustrated by Bush et al. (1972), who analyzed the New York State phenylketonuria screening program and showed that, while the program costs $38,000.00 per detected case, the resulting treatment averts institutionalization costs of $50,000.00 per case. By contrast, screening programs for sicklemia, lacking means for either prevention or treatment, have been judged a fiasco (Bylinsky, 1974).

Experts in diabetes concede that there is no evidence that early diagnosis improves the course of the disease. Meanwhile, the premature diagnosis of diabetes can be 'very detrimental' to the patient who may lose insurance and encounter job restrictions (Foster, 1975).

Several formulae have been proposed for predicting the yield and cost effectiveness of health screening, the most comprehensive being those of Emlet (1968). In addition, multiphasic screening multiplies the problems of cost, effectiveness and justification by the number of parameters being evaluated.

Pollard (1972) calls attention to the magnitude of statistical problems involved in evaluating the benefits of multiphasic screening. He mentions particularly:

1. The number of persons required to be screened to produce significant results when only 1% or so show true positive results is very large.

2. The number of years that persons with true positive results must remain under observation in order to detect morbidity, and particularly mortality, differentials is considerable.

3. The difficulties of obtaining appropriate control groups and maintaining them as controls, i.e. preventing them from obtaining examinations, etc. are very great.

4. The results of screening are not independent of the type of population screened or the level of medical care received by the population.

5. Care must be taken to ensure in the statistical analysis that the earlier detection of disease by screening (say 5 years earlier than when symptoms have appeared) does not lead to a false deduction of longer survival.

6. 'Check-ups' must be distinguished from routine screenings. A much higher incidence of true positive results would be expected in the former.

7. The benefits of screening depend on the regularity and quality of subsequent care. Some machinery is necessary to see that this is assured.

All things considered, at least from the point of view of cost effectiveness, many would agree with Burrows (1972) that 'multiphasic biochemical screening in the current form is probably not justified for the routine study of outpatients'.

Laboratory testing in a diagnostic setting

Laboratory testing involving persons with symptoms and signs of disease has other clearly defined objectives, as shown in Table 6. In this setting, we are concerned less with the inherent 'technical' reliability of a test and more with

TABLE 6

Objectives of testing in a diagnostic setting

1. To diagnose disease and define its extent and severity
2. To identify etiologic agents or factors
3. To assess functional impairment
4. To evaluate the patient's capacity to survive rigorous therapy (functional reserve)

'diagnostic' validity and effectiveness, or value (Werner et al., 1973). When more than one laboratory test might be used to discern a suspected disease, it is of interest to select that test which is most cost effective. Werner et al. present formulae relating the costs of doing the test, the cost of false positive results, the cost of false negative results, and the cost of late results with an estimate of disease prevalence in the target population and the trade-off between sensitivity and specificity to arrive at a mathematical value representing the total cost of the test. By performing similar analyses of all available alternative procedures, relative cost effectiveness can be compared among similar tests.

In most hospital settings, however, the practical problems of the cost effective use of laboratory facilities concerns questions of over- or underutilization of test curricula, rather than discrimination among similar tests. LaCombe (1973) has proposed that house staff should order tests only if the result will benefit the patient or change his therapy, contribute to education or medical knowledge, or is likely to 'discover' something.

Williams (1972) discusses and illustrates the value of developing normative standards for retrospective evaluation of the utilization of laboratory facilities in the diagnosis and treatment of defined disease entities or clinical problems. Her studies of laboratory tests for 133 male patients treated in Veteran Administration Hospitals in the U.S. with a diagnosis of lung cancer, showed a greater prevalence of under-testing than over-testing. This unexpected result is explained by the normative standard's requirement for an array of procedures to establish a data base and to monitor progress, requirements which can be fulfilled readily only when multichannel analyzers for battery testing in hematology and chemistry are available.

A College of American Pathologists Committee has been assigned the task of developing a rational approach to laboratory testing. The Committee to Develop Guidelines for the Appropriate Utilization of Laboratory Procedures (Cole, 1975, personal communication) has classified laboratory tests into several categories for the purpose of defining the most appropriate, and therefore the most cost effective, selection of laboratory tests to solve clinical problems. The categories are shown in Table 7.

TABLE 7

Test categories

---

1. Tests related to general inflammation, injury and repair
2. Tests of general metabolic function
3. Organ system tests:
   a Tests of injury, inflammation and repair
   b Tests of metabolic function
4. Etiology-related tests
5. Therapeutic monitors

The first three categories are subdivided into primary, secondary and tertiary test groupings. Primary tests are usually available in general laboratories and some may be automated. Secondary tests are ones usually available in large laboratories and are indicated in order to define abnormalities revealed in primary tests or suggested by high clinical suspicion. Tertiary tests are generally exotic procedures performed in reference laboratories and needed for special problems.

As a result of its evaluation of primary tests pertinent to arriving at a diagnosis in the categories above and establishing essential baselines for subsequent monitoring of therapy, the committee has concluded that the most effective scheme for minimizing elapsed time for diagnosis and extraneous testing, evaluating the extent of disease and functional reserve, and delineating baselines consists of the multiparameter chemical and hematologic tests presently available from screening instruments plus appropriate tests of electrolytes and basic urinalysis and serology. Thus, running a comprehensive laboratory 'profile' on patients being evaluated for definitive diagnosis and therapy at the time of the initial visit, or admission to a hospital, saves valuable time and hospitalization expense, and thus is the most cost effective approach to laboratory testing in the diagnostic setting. In addition, rescheduling the laboratory work to run tests as soon after the initial patient contact as possible may save a day or more of valuable and expensive time (Dorsey, 1970).

Laboratory testing in a therapeutic setting

Laboratory testing in a therapeutic setting has relevant objectives, as shown in Table 8. Laboratory testing for critically ill or injured, metabolically unstable patients must be much more concerned with effectiveness in terms of minimal delay in testing and reporting, and proper selection of tests than with cost

TABLE 8

Objectives of testing in the therapeutic setting

1. To monitor the internal environment
2. To assess response to therapy
3. To evaluate end results
4. To evaluate therapeutic effectiveness
5. To assess alternative modalities

conservation. It costs less to run tests in batches on automated equipment, but the patient may be dead by the time the result is available.

Even in this setting, however, cost can be minimized by appropriate test selection and timing. Why run a complete blood count, when a hemoglobin gives all the information needed? Why run a SMA 12/60 daily, if an enzyme is all you need?

Conclusion

1. To evaluate cost effectiveness we must include all related costs and define 'effective'.

2. The definition of 'effective' varies with the testing mode.

3. Cost effective testing in the public health setting is determined by extrapolation of a limited number of tests to benefit large population groups, with important reductions in morbidity and mortality rates.

4. The cost effectiveness of testing in the screening mode is vitally dependent on the availability, effectiveness and cost of preventive or remedial measures. The effective yield of screening programs is determined by the sensitivity and specificity of the test and decreases rapidly with decreasing incidence of the disease.

5. The cost effectiveness of testing in the diagnostic mode is determined by conserving time and expense in establishing the diagnosis, evaluating the extent of disease and degree of functional impairment, and in determining the ability of the patient to survive rigorous therapy, together with establishing required baselines for monitoring, thus constituting a legitimate role for multiphasic screening.

6. Cost effective therapeutic monitoring must emphasize effectiveness more than cost, but elimination of mindless repetition of extraneous tests can still conserve resources.

References

Burrows, S. (1972): *J. med. Soc. New Jersey, 69,* 919.

Bush, J. W., Chen, M. M. and Patrick, D. L. (1972): In: *Health Status Indexes, Proceedings of a Conference Conducted by Health Services Research.* Editor: R. L. Berg. Hospital Research and Educational Trust.

Bylinsky, G. (1974): *Fortune,* 148.

Collen, M. F., Dales, L. G., Friedman, D., Flagle, C. D., Feldman, R. and Siegelaub, A. B. (1973): *Preventive Med., 2,* 236.

Collen, M. D., Feldman, R., Siegelaub, A. B. and Crawford, D. (1970): *New Engl. J. Med., 283,* 459.

Dorsey, D. B. (1970): *Pathologist, 24,* 113.

Emlet Jr, H. E., (Ed.) (1968): In: *The Engineering Research Conference on Physical Parameters in Multiphasic Screening.* Analytic Services, Inc.

Foster, D. W. (1975): *Int. med. News, 8,* 3.

La Combe, M. A. (1973): *Resident and Staff Physician, 19,* 46.

Mechanic, D. (1975): *Amer. J. Publ. Health, 65,* 241.

Paulus, H. E., Coutts, A., Calabro, J. J. and Klineberg, J. R. (1970): *J. Amer. med. Ass., 211,* 277.

Peery, T. M. (1975): *Amer. J. clin. Path., 63,* 453.

Pollard, A. H. (1972): *Med. J. Austr., 2,* 1025.

Werner, M., Brooks, S. H. and Welte, R. (1973): *Hum. Path., 4,* 17.

Williams, M. J. (1972) *Pathologist, 26,* 263.

Wolf Jr, G. A. (1972): *Hospitals, 46,* 65.

Hospital laboratory planning in the future

Lorentz Eldjarn

Institute of Clinical Biochemistry, Rikshospitalet, University of Oslo, Norway

Around the world the design of hospital laboratories varies tremendously. It reflects not only the taste and imagination of the architect and the effects of climate and local building regulations, but also the multitude of medical laboratory specialties, the desire of strong personalities to measure their local kingdom in square feet, the slowness with which claims and demands are adapted to the changing state of the art, and the demands of the staff of the clinical department for access to laboratory space. Laboratory activities have grown tremendously during the last few decades, both in volume and in sophistication. Hospital laboratories therefore also to some extent reflect the technical development and economy of the population in question. In most hospitals the laboratory activities take place in rooms and corridors constructed for quite different purposes, and often resemble an intricate maze.

My views on the planning of hospital laboratories are of course strongly influenced by the situation in Scandinavia, which has a reasonable socio-economic level, free hospital medicare, governmental control of essentially all hospitals, and permanent medical staffing of these institutions. In our part of the world, opposing views are held concerning hospital laboratory planning. However, the main ideas set out here have been presented in a collegial report (Eldjarn and Lingjaerde, 1970) and have been to varying degrees implemented in many modern Scandinavian hospital buildings.

This discussion will deal in particular with the general non-teaching hospital of 500-1000 beds serving a population of a few hundred thousand. Conditions in a university hospital with extensive education and research responsibilities may be more complex and call for a greater subdivision of laboratory activities. It should be stressed, however, that the design of the latter should be considered the exception and not necessarily the goal and ideal of the regional general hospital. In my opinion the routine laboratory activities at the university hospital level should in principle be organized along the same lines as in the non-teaching hospital. As will appear later, our own University Department of Clinical Biochemistry at Rikshospitalet, the University Hospital of Oslo, has been organized according to the ideas to be presented. The distinctive feature of the hospital is that all departments have access to research facilities.

The appearance of the future hospital laboratory depends primarily on its subdivision and functional pattern, and only secondarily on the architectural and instrumental design. It is my conviction that the planning of new hospital laboratories should start with a reappraisal of their purpose, aim and function in modern medicine. In this process it is necessary for the medical profession to rid itself of the heavy load of prejudices from the past and to mould its thinking according to present demands and intelligent guesswork about the future.

The object of laboratory medicine is to bridge bench-side and bed-side medicine

Modern hospitals are built on the idea that certain areas of medicine, for economic as well as professional reasons, should be included under one guidance and in one departmental structure. Thus, despite the fact that all medical doctors may possess an ophthalmoscope and include a judgement of the fundus oculi in their investigation of the patient, the Department of Ophthalmology is still considered to be the main body in charge of ophthalmological problems. The same holds true for departments of gynecology and obstetrics, otolaryngology, surgery and internal medicine. In clinical medicine this subdivision largely merges with the existing system of medical specialties.

However, in laboratory medicine this is not the case. In most hospitals the prevailing view is that for economic reasons some routine investigations should be centralized in a report- and result-producing laboratory department. The bed-side use of these results is, however, solely a matter for the clinician. Furthermore, the more specialized laboratory work is considered to be the responsibility of the clinician. As a consequence many clinical departments run various types of independent laboratory set-ups. These activities are largely related to chemical pathology, but histology, cytology and microbiology may also be involved. This development can most clearly be seen from the distribution of technical laboratory personnel within the hospital: it is generally found that $\frac{1}{4}$ or less are in the laboratory department proper. In particular, the department of chemical pathology may suffer from this structure and become merely an analytical assembly-line occupied with automation and data processing.

Several arguments may be put forward in favour of independent 'special' laboratories attached to clinical departments. Some branches of clinical medicine have an obvious need for close contact with laboratory activites. Thus, clinical physiology, involving heart catheterization, the evaluation of kidney and liver function or intestinal mucosa biopsies, calls for close contact with laboratory facilities. Similarly, it is easy to understand that a department of pediatrics may want to exclude possible inherited metabolic defects. Past experience shows that much good research has come out of the existing system. The fact that the person who asks for the tests is also responsible for the technical performance and evaluation of the results considerably reduces the number of complaints concerning efficiency and quality.

The structure of hospital laboratory activities described is rapidly changing. The tremendous growth in the activities and significance of laboratory medicine in recent decades has caused an obvious imbalance in the existing system. A large proportion of the tests performed on patients are probably unnecessary, and the full significance of those that are necessary is not always appreciated. Extensive technical improvements and the growth of automation have for a decade led laboratory medicine astray. The increase in output has created a 'supermarket' atmosphere which deters medical doctors from starting on a career in this discipline (Astrup, 1975), and provoked a *Lancet* editorial headed: 'Chemical pathology–any future?' (*Lancet,* 1975, *1,* 1327). This failure in recruiting also applies to chemists with a science education. Of particular significance in bringing about a change is the fact that the modern hospital laboratory requires considerable space, is complex and expensive to build, calls for frequent changes and readjustments and requires expensive equipment and personnel. It is being realized – not least by the hospital owners – that to make the most of these resources, the hospital laboratory must be well organized, and that well trained personnel of various categories are needed. Among these are the medical laboratory specialists, who should be in charge of and coordinate the use of the facilities.

What is needed is a reappraisal of the aims of laboratory medicine. The technical production of results should become the means and not the measure. On the other hand, this production is too complicated and too expensive to be distributed all over the hospital according to the varying interests of colleagues. The future goal of laboratory medicine should first and foremost be to form a bridge between basic biochemical and biological science on the one hand and bed-side medicine on the other. The gap between the appearance of up-to-date biological information and its application in the care of patients is steadily increasing. The amount of laboratory information available on the diagnosis and treatment of patients is expanding rapidly. It is well known that clinicians encounter great difficulty in including this new knowledge in the daily routine. In my view, the medical staff of the laboratory have a particular responsibility in this respect. Their basic medical education combined with their thorough training in biology and chemical pathology make them particularly suited for bridging this gap. It is essential, however, that the planning of the future laboratory allows this function to be fulfilled.

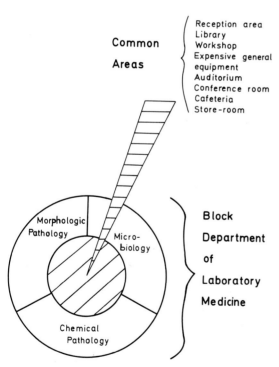

Fig. 1. Main laboratory of the block department of laboratory medicine.

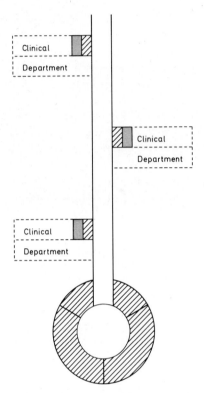

Block Department of Laboratory Medicine

Fig. 2. The block department of laboratory medicine should comprise the main laboratory area as well as primary laboratories strategically placed in the clinical departments. The laboratories of clinical departments for physiological investigations on patients should be in or at the primary laboratories.

Laboratory medicine should be organized as one hospital block department

In planning a future hospital laboratory, all routine laboratory activities should be united in one organization, a hospital block department. Its physical and organizational structure should not only satisfy the needs of clinicians for laboratory contact and of laboratory medical staff for clinical contact, but also take into account the extensive overlap between the various areas of laboratory medicine.

In my judgement the purpose and function of the future hospital laboratory should be planned according to the general structure given in Figures 1 and 2.

The block department of laboratory medicine consists of a main laboratory area plus detached small 'primary laboratories' strategically sited among the clinical departments.

The department should be divided into three main sections: morphological pathology, chemical pathology, and microbiology. This division should be only partial because several functions should be combined, e.g. the reception area for patients and for samples, office space, library, animal house, workshop, and expensive technical and chemical equipment.

The primary laboratories should serve as centers for sample collection and provide laboratory space for simpler blood and urine tests when centralization does not offer any advantage.

Efficient transport systems for patients and for samples should be constructed between the primary laboratories and the reception area of the main laboratory. Similarly, an efficient and rapid reporting system from the laboratory to the clinical departments must be included.

The primary laboratories and their location in the clinical departments present the staff of the department of laboratory medicine with an excellent opportunity to secure the necessary contact with the staff of the clinical department. I believe that the medical staff of the department of laboratory medicine should spend part of the working day in various clinical departments, particularly those of internal medicine and pediatrics and the intensive care units. Conversely, the legitimate need of the staff of the clinical departments for laboratory contact should be fulfilled in the primary laboratories or in adjacent clinical investigation rooms.

In most instances the hospital laboratory must be planned to serve not only the in-patients but also the surrounding community on an out-patient basis. In our part of the world this often represents 50% of the work.

In order to fulfill the above requirements the department of laboratory medicine should be situated at or near ground level in the hospital block, or possibly in a separate laboratory building. The area needed for the laboratory department in the type of hospital under consideration in Norway is reckoned to be in the order of 3000 to 6000 m^2 effective floor space (or approximately 5000 to 9000 m^2 gross). The distribution of this space between the various activities should be based on the real and expected workload and not on traditional reluctance to change. Thus, the department of chemical pathology (including nuclear medicine and the blood transfusion unit) usually occupies about 50% of the space available.

Hospital laboratory planning and the existing laboratory specialties

Hospital laboratory planning is strongly influenced by the existing system of laboratory specialties. The urge of each primary specialty to establish an independent department second to none seems irresistible. It should be stressed, however, that such consequences were seldom foreseen when new specialties were created.

The present system of medical specialties has developed gradually over nearly 100 years. During this time the arguments put forward for the creation of a new specialty have changed considerably, at least in Norway. In the beginning, a specialist had to observe certain professional rules before being allowed to advertise himself as a specialist. Later, when social security systems were introduced, the problem of increasing fees also had to be taken into consideration. During the last 30-40 years the main argument used has been that a particular area of medicine has become so vast and complicated that it is impossible for one person to master it all. New specialties were also advocated in order to further the development of a particular area of medicine (i.e. research) and to attract gifted colleagues to that field. Although never stated openly, personal prestige and the search for an identity may have been strong motives.

There is a clear difference between the development of clinical and laboratory specialties. Following the establishment of the large clinical specialties early in this century, further specialization took place relatively late and resulted in subspecialties which involve additional special education after the full training programme of the primary or basic specialty (see Fig. 3). In the case of laboratory specialties, however, a tendency to branching appeared very early in most countries and resulted in a maze of usually more or less unrelated and self-sufficient educational systems of fully independent disciplines (Fig. 3). Thus, in addition to the three main branches of morphological pathology, chemical pathology and microbiology, there are a great number of other specialties: haematology, clinical physiology, endocrinology, nuclear medicine, clinical immunology, virology, parasitology, forensic pathology, immune haematology and blood transfusion, clinical pharmacology and clinical neurophysiology. As is so often the case in medicine, the system of classification varies, being in part functional, according to organ systems, in part biochemical, and in part technical. As a result there is a great deal of overlapping.

In the course of the last decade it has become increasingly evident that the structure of our health care systems and the planning of our hospitals is to an increasing extent being determined by the number and types of medical specialties. Because of the pronounced and complete subdivision of laboratory medicine, many countries are confronted with a disparity between the existing

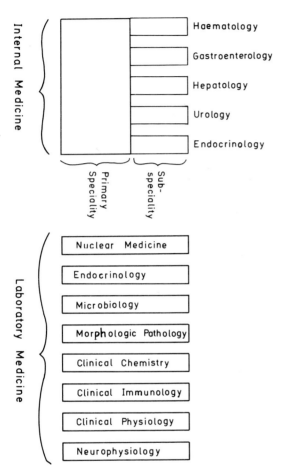

Fig. 3. The difference in independence and educational structure of clinical and laboratory medical specialties.

and forseeable needs of health care planning and the type of personnel educated.

It seems clear that a close relation between existing laboratory specialties and the planning of health care will always exist. In Norway this was realized when our Medical Association recently accepted the following definition of a medical specialty, as proposed by a working committee (Eldjarn and Holand, 1973): 'A medical specialty is a sector of medicine which is delineated because it is necessary for patient care within the planned national system of health service'. This definition stresses that the evaluation of a possible new medical specialty should be governed by implementation and not by research and development. It also implies that the creation of a medical specialty is not only a matter for the medical profession. Other bodies will obviously have responsibilities for evaluating the positive and negative effects of a new subdivision on the planned national system of health care. Such a definition also recognizes differences in medical specialties between countries, depending on geography, economy and the spectrum of diseases to be combatted. The argument that a medical specialty should be created because it already exists in a number of other countries will therefore be of dubious value.

It is my conviction that despite the tremendous resistance to change, a number of countries should reappraise their system of medical laboratory specialties. In most countries there is a well defined need for three main laboratory specialties: morphological pathology, chemical pathology and microbiology. It seems reasonable that some of the other existing laboratory specialties should be redistributed between these main specialties, whereas others should reappear in due course as subspecialties.

The implementation of some of these ideas in our Department of Clinical Biochemistry at Rikshospitalet, the University Hospital of Oslo

Our hospital has about 1000 beds distributed between 15 clinical departments of various kinds. In 1960 there was a total of 33 independent laboratories of clinical pathology, of which our Department of Clinical Biochemistry was one. In the course of the last 15 years we have tried to gradually develop our own department to cover routine aspects of chemical pathology in the broader sense of the term. We started out with a small analytical central laboratory of 17 technicians, one chemist and two M.D.s. The growth has been gradual, since no new laboratory field has been included until it was requested by those formerly responsible. Major activities in chemical pathology are still covered by special units under the guidance of clinicians in internal medicine or pediatrics, and our department includes only 50% of the technical staff of the hospital active in chemical pathology work.

Our present organizational structure is shown in Figure 4. A total of 7 primary laboratories in the organization form the basis for blood sampling and simple haematological and urine tests which are our responsibility. These primary laboratories also serve as centres of contact between the clinical and laboratory departments.

The main area of the department is organized as shown in Figure 4. We have tried to follow biochemical principles of division as against the organ-orientated

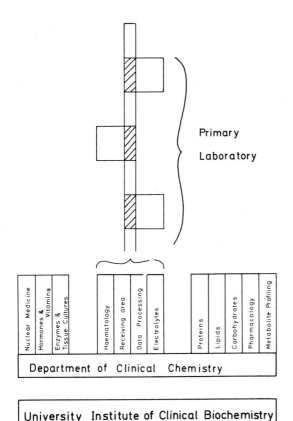

Fig. 4. The organizational structure of the Chemical Pathology Department, Rikshospitalet, the University Hospital of Oslo, Norway.

system of the clinicians. We believe that confrontation between these two systems leads to improved cooperation.

The workload and responsibilities of our routine department soon resulted in an efficient but strained unit continuously subject to growth and development. Being a university department with obvious research and educational responsibilities, we therefore in 1961 founded the University Institute of Clinical Biochemistry alongside the routine department. Apart from providing pre- and postgraduate medical education, this Institute, in close cooperation with the routine department, soon established efficient research activities on problems in chemical pathology.

In this set-up for routine and research activities in chemical pathology about 18 medical doctors and one chemist are currently working full-time: 5 in permanent positions at the Institute; 6 as research fellows paid by various humanitarian organizations; 2 in permanent positions in the section of nuclear medicine; and 5 in the other routine sections. For educational purposes considerable circulation takes place. Also, nearly all are pursuing research activities at the Institute. The aim is for about 1/3 of the total working hours of the medical staff to be spent in cooperation with the clinical departments, about 1/3 in supervising the various sections of the routine laboratory, and about 1/3 in developmental work and research. Our technical staff consists of approximately 70 'physiochemists', a devoted group of personnel specifically trained in special schools for work in modern chemical pathology.

Architectural and technical design of future hospital laboratories

The architectural and technical design of hospital laboratories is primarily dependent on the subdivision and functional structure described. Other important factors are rules and regulation for building activities pertaining to the country, security of the working personnel, possible risks to adjacent departments and pollution of the surrounding district. In most countries detailed regulations exist with regard to building construction, fire precautions, industrial hygiene, electrical installations, temperature, light and humidity, handling of gasses under pressure, storage and work with inflammable or explosive materials, radioactivity, etc. All these factors are of prime importance in hospital planning, but they are beyond the scope of the present discussion. A number of useful publications on this subject may be consulted (Dehlholm et al., 1961; Erler et al., 1962; Lewis, 1962; Nuffield Foundation, 1961; Schramm, 1960; *Hospital Management,* 1971).

However, there is one prime and major requirement for any future hospital laboratory design – flexibility. In the last twenty-five years we have seen continuous expansion and remodelling of laboratory medicine due to unforseeable progress. It seems obvious that this development will continue. Despite all attempts at intelligent projections about the future, unexpected changes must be anticipated. The basic laboratory design should therefore be large, open spaces in which walls and technical supplies can easily be changed and installed wherever needed.

National advisory boards for hospital laboratory planning

The design of a hospital is a two-step process: firstly the users formulate the purpose, aim and function of the planned laboratories; secondly, the architect and his consultants propose a solution within the framework of the hospital and economy involved. Throughout the planning phase there should be a continuous flow of information between users and planners.

Usually a local building committee is appointed. Here the local medical departmental heads formulate the needs and wishes of the users. This group takes on a tremendous responsibility considering the vast investment involved in a modern hospital building and the fact that it will be in use for generations. In fact, the local user is planning not for himself, but for his successor.

Realizing this, over 10 years ago the Norwegian Society for Clinical Chemistry appointed an Advisory Board for Hospital Laboratory Construction with the aim of relieving local colleagues of some of the responsibilities. Since then nearly all plans for new hospital laboratories in our country have passed this Board, which consists of 5 experienced chemical pathologists and one hospital architect.

To bring about an organized approach to the design of future hospital laboratories it is advocated that an international expert meeting produce guidelines for these activities and that the professions involved appoint advisory boards on a national level for hospital laboratory construction. This might prove helpful in future hospital laboratory planning.

Summary

There is tremendous diversity in the design of hospital laboratories around the world. This makes it difficult to discuss the planning of hospital laboratories in the future without stating the obvious to some, the unwanted to others and the impossible to a few.

The planning of the future hospital laboratory depends above all on a reappraisal of the aim and function of future laboratory medicine. The tremendous growth and expansion in this area of medicine in recent decades has resulted in an overvaluation of technical perfection. This has occurred at the cost of interpretation in relation to the individual patient and implementation of the activities in the system of health care. The result has been a damaging subdivision of laboratory medicine into a maze of independent specialties based on technical subtleties. In addition, more routine laboratory medical work is usually being performed in a large number of small laboratories run by clinicians than in the department of laboratory medicine proper.

A reappraisal of laboratory medicine should result in hospital laboratories reducing the number of independent laboratory units and creating a laboratory block department. This department should have separate primary laboratories situated among the clinical departments, which will also serve to promote the necessary contact between the medical personnel in the clinical and laboratory departments.

It is realized that the conservative character of the medical profession makes such changes difficult. One possible approach would be to redefine the system of medical specialties. Another, less effective, approach would be to adopt the principle that various medical laboratory specialists should work as section leaders within the same organizational laboratory structure.

References

Astrup, P. (1975): *Clin. Chem.,* in press.

Dehlholm, B., Djurtoft, R., Nielsen, K. E. and Niepoort, P. (ed.) (1961): *Laboratorier.* Teknisk Forlag, Copenhagen (In Danish).

Eldjarn, L. and Holand, H. (1973): *T. norske Lageforen., 9,* 617.

Eldjarn, L. and Lingjaerde, P. (1970): *Nord. Med., 84,* 947.

Erler, H., Schmincke, W. and Weber, G. (1962): *Das stationäre und ambulante Gesundheitswesen. Planung, Organisation, Bau und Betrieb, Vol. 2,* pp. 1-71. VEB Verlag Volk und Gesundheit, Berlin.

Hospital Management (1971): *Modern British Medical Laboratories* (Suppl. pp. 77-112). Whitehall Press Ltd., London.

Lewis, H. F. (ed.) (1962): *Laboratory Planning for Chemistry and Chemical Engineering.* Reinhold Publishing Co., New York.

The Nuffield Foundation Division for Architectural Studies (1961): *The Design of Research Laboratories.* Oxford University Press, London.

Schramm, W. (1960): *Chemische und biologische Laboratorien. Planung. Bau und Einrichtung.* Verlag Chemie GmbH, Weinheim.

An audio-response communications system for order entry and result retrieval in an automated computerized clinical laboratory*

A. E. Rappoport, W. D. Gennaro and R. E. Berquist

The Youngstown Hospital Association, Youngstown, Ohio, U.S.A.

In previous publications (Rappoport et al., 1964, 1967, 1968; Rappoport and Rappoport, 1970; Rappoport, 1971, 1973), we reported the initial development of the computerized laboratory information system of The Youngstown Hospital Association in Youngstown, Ohio, U.S.A. It consisted of an on-line, automated, electronic instrument, data acquisition system (IBM 1080) for calculating test results and associated with positive specimen identification. This was linked off-line to an IBM 360/30 computer which daily generated updated patient, cumulative reports containing automated, semiautomated, and manual test results from all laboratory sections including pathology and microbiology.

Later (Rappoport and Gennaro, 1974), we presented a review of the increasingly sophisticated and expanded, soft- and hardware systems configuration then available in our laboratory. We discussed important operational concepts and criteria for selection of computer systems, including the evaluation of their cost effectiveness, impact on technologist acceptance and productivity, and speed of operating. We emphasized the improvement obtained in the analyt-

* This project was supported by Grant Number R18 HS 00060 from the National Center for Health Services Research, HRA, PHS.

ical and documentation subsystems which have contributed to greatly enhanced accuracy, precision, and economy of testing.

Subsequently, to close the communication loop between nursing stations and physicians' offices and the laboratory, to order tests and to obtain complete test results, we created DIVOTS (Direct Input Voice Output Telephone System), an on-line, audio-response, laboratory communication system. This is now completely operational in our North Side Unit (Lewis, 1975; Keller, 1975; Rappoport et al., 1975a), and used for test order entry and result retrieval.

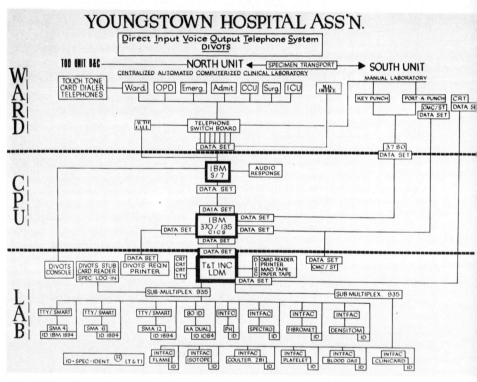

Fig. 1. Flow Chart showing the telephone connections to the IBM System/7 possessing the audio-response unit. This computer communicates with the IBM 370 containing the patient's data base. Note the analytic instruments and SPEC-IDENTS® connected on-line to the laboratory computer (LDM) for data reduction, specimen identification, and automatic, on-line transmission to the 370 of results which then become immediately available to DIVOTS for communication to physicians.

The computerized laboratory

To comprehend DIVOTS, a brief description of the functional and structural characteristics of our data acquisition system and laboratory information and communication system is necessary (Fig. 1).

The total hospital information system, which will not be described further, is centered around an IBM 370/135 computer with 386 K operating under CICS/DOS. This contains every patient's medical data bases accumulated during their entire hospital stay as well as a multitude of administrative professional pro-programs and terminals.

The data acquisition system consists of a dedicated laboratory computer, the T and T, Inc. Laboratory Data Manager (LDM), possessing a Data General NOVA 1200 computer, and other devices (printer, CRT, card reader). The LDM receives and processes simultaneously all the analog and digital signals from 15 automated and semiautomated electronic instruments which have been outfitted with appropriate interfaces and sample identification devices (SPEC-IDENT®) capable of reading human- and machine-readable keypunched stub-cards attached to the Vacutainer® blood samples.

After data reduction, the LDM merges the test results with the stub-card identification number. Manual test results (e.g. urinalysis) are entered by CRT, Diskette, Key- or Port-A-Punch cards. The LDM transmits these results by telephone line and data sets (4800 Baud) to the IBM 370, where they are filed automatically within each patient's master file. Free, narrative reports (e.g. surgical pathology, EKG, microbiology) are prepared and transmitted to the 370 by the Communicating Magnetic Card Selectric Typewriter (Rappoport et al., 1975b).

An Interim Ward Report is printed at 13.00 hours daily for each nursing station listing all patients and their available test results up to that hour. The cumulative Patient Summary Report, listing all completed results for that day and the past 6 days, is updated and printed each evening at 18.00 hours. This report permits chronologic comparison of serial values of the same test on horizontal lines while groups of tests relevant to the clinical disease or substance being studied are listed vertically (Fig. 2).

DIVOTS

DIVOTS serves to make these results available to physicians immediately on completion of the test and thus to expedite the doctor's decision-making process. DIVOTS' hardware consists of an IBM System/7 computer (S/7) with 24

```
                                                        PAGE  2
                                                        TIME 19.03
                   THE YOUNGSTOWN HOSPITAL ASSOCIATION
         NORTH UNIT PATIENT CUMULATIVE REPORT  DATE 03/18/75   PROV DIAG-CORONARY

1NORTH WEST   1106-A   8126593   AGE 49 M   ADM DATE 03/15/75   PROV DIAG-CORONARY
KUNKEL F MD

                             SATURDAY   SUNDAY     MONDAY     TUESDAY
                             03/15/75   03/16/75   03/17/75   03/18/75
              HOSPITAL DAY   1          2          3          4

CO2 CONT PLASMA 25-32 MEQ/L  26.1
PH PLASMA VENOUS  7.32-7.45  7.42
GLUCOSE FASTING 70-110 MGM%  122
CHOLESTEROL  150-250 MGM%    200        *
TPIGLYCERIDE  50-150 MGM%    115
SGOT         5-40 MU/ML      41         * 30       22
LDH        100-225 MU/ML     171        149        169
LDH ISOENZYME PATTERN
         INTERPRETATION      NORM       NORM       NORM
CREAT PHOS KIN 25-145 MU/ML  105        123        107
SEROLOGY
VDRL                         NON REACT
VIROLOGY
COMPLEMENT FIXATION-RESP
    INFLUENZA A                                               1/16
    PARA INFLUENZA 1                                          NEG
    PARA INFLUENZA 2                                          NEG
    PARA INFLUENZA 3                                          NEG
    ADENOVIRUS                                                1/4
    RESPIRATORY SYNCYTIAL                                     NEG
EKG INTERPRETATION     03/15   INFERIOR MYOCARDIAL INFARCTION AGE UNDETERMINED.
                               POSSIBLE---COMPLETE RIGHT BUNDLE BRANCH BLOCK
EKG INTERPRETATION     03/16   INFERIOR MYOCARDIAL INFARCTION AGE UNDETERMINED. POSSIBLE---2ND
                               DEGREE AV BLOCK MOBITZ TYPE I  2 TO 1 OR 3 TO 1 RESPONSE--- SINUS
                               BRADYCARDIA
CHEMISTRY INTERPRETATION 03/15  RESULTS MAY BE AFFECTED BY IV
```

Fig. 2. Cumulative patient summary report. Note the horizontal arrangement of several days' test data permitting comparative evaluation of results. Test results are listed in a vertical clustering relevant to specific diseases, organs, or substances, i.e. electrolytes, metabolic products. Note the inclusion of EKG results on the same report to help evaluate and correlate with cardiac enzyme and other studies.

K, a fixed disk for programs and a removable disk possessing the digitized, audio-response vocabulary of 850 words appropriate for medical and laboratory use. This includes all the letters of the alphabet, numbers up to a million, selected Greek letters and symbols, chemical units, general administrative and technical words, the names of all tests and many descriptive words necessary to report verbally diagnostic and numeric results generated by the various sections of our total laboratory, which performs a wide variety of anatomic pathology and clinical pathology tests.

These words had been recorded previously on high quality magnetic tape on equipment in the local TV/radio station. The dictated words were digitized in the IBM Phono-laboratory and transferred to S/7 disk.

DIVOTS operates from any Touch-Tone (T-T) telephone within the hospital, the physician's office or home or anywhere else in the world. If a standard T-T phone is not available, an ordinary phone may be converted by a small, battery-operated accessory T-T 'pad' attached to the mouthpiece of the handset (Fig. 3).

Communicating with the S/7 by appropriate Data Sets are three internal, hospital telephones lines connected to the automatic hospital switchboard and 1 external, private commercial line which bypasses the switchboard. The S/7 is coupled to the 370 by another Data Set (WE202R). The programs governing S/7-370 communications and the location addresses for all the digitized words are located in the 370.

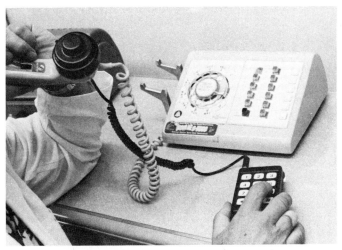

Fig. 3. Note a Touch-Tone pad with card dialer accessory attached to the mouthpiece of a conventional rotary phone. This is used to input coded numerical instructions and to hear patient's test results from physicians' offices or homes.

Order entry

DIVOTS is operated as follows. On admission, the patient's complete demographic data are entered by a clerk in the Admitting Office into the 370 computer
through a CRT. The patient is assigned a unique hospital number and receives
an embossed telephone Dialer-Card containing his punched-in hospital number

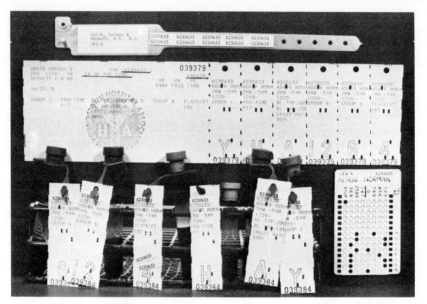

Fig. 4. This demonstrates the punched Dial-a-Card (lower right) and patient identification wrist band bearing the pressure labels imprinted with his hospital number. Note the
requisition (top) printed in the laboratory by the 370. The left-hand portion is the audit
trail, file copy. It gives the clinical (admitting) diagnosis. Note the repeat printing of the
specimen number (039379) under the printed number by the computer which merges it
with the hospital number (8230633). Thus, the punched stub-cards attached to the tubes,
when read by the SPEC-IDENT®, identifies the patient from whom the specimen was
obtained. Observe the location of the pressure labels above the computer printed number
on the stub-card.

A duplicate requisition has been burst and the variously identified (SMA 12, 6, 4, etc.)
stub-cards have been attached to tubes containing specimens which will be tested for the
procedures printed on each stub-card and file copy.

There are two extra labels on the Stub-card 4 (EDTA tube for hematology). One label
will be attached to the slide to be stained for the differential count and the other is to be
attached to a special differential Port-A-Punch card for reporting the result. Both serve
to insure correctness of specimen and patient identification even in a manual test.

and a human-readable identification wrist-band bearing removable pressure labels imprinted with that number (Fig. 4).

When the patient arrives on the nursing station with the physician's orders for tests, the nurse initiates a telephone call (Extension 461) to the S/7, which responds with a high pitched 'beep' and says, 'Please enter request', which is done on the T-T phone.

Test request is achieved by two codes: No. 1 for beginners, and No. 2 for experienced personnel. In Code 1, the S/7 maintains a dialog with the clerk, telling him the next step to take in using DIVOTS. When employing Code 2, DIVOTS merely responds to and confirms each successive input with a high-pitched beep indicating that the clerk is correct and should proceed automatically to the next step. If an input error is made, DIVOTS states 'Error' and instructs how to correct.

The next instruction is 'Enter Patient Number'. The clerk inserts the patient's Dialer Card into the telephone or enters the number manually by T-T. The S/7 relays the number to the 370, which locates the patient's file and returns appropriate instructions to the S/7 to spell the name, heard by the clerk within 2-3 seconds after input (Fig. 5).

To verify the accuracy of the patient's identification, S/7 requests the patient's ward number and checks it against the 370 file; the clerk is then required to enter

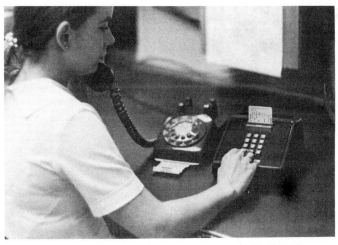

Fig. 5. On nursing stations, there are Touch-Tone, Card-Dialer accessories modifying the conventional phones. Note a patient's Dialer-Card inserted into the device while the Nurse enters test codes. Observe the pull-out DIVOT test directory containing test codes below rotary phone.

the time of day that the test was requested by the physician since it measures the elapsed times between the various steps in the total test path.

In the next step, DIVOTS requests order of the desired tests. The clerk enters appropriate 4-digit codes for each procedure obtained from a Test Directory. The name is verified audibly immediately and contributes to the correctness of the order. If an error is made, the test may be deleted by operating the asterisk key.

The nine most frequently requested tests or profiles (e.g. hemoglobin, SMA, etc.) in our laboratory can be ordered by entering only a single digit on the T-T pad. Nine special instructions such as 'urgent', 'preoperative', 'special collection time', 'next day', etc. are also entered by a single digit and are confirmed audibly. Upon completion of the total transaction for each patient, DIVOTS states 'Order accepted'. The clerk may now order tests for other patients or she may terminate the process and 'hang up'. Using Code 2 materially shortens the transaction time since there is no dialog and DIVOTS does not instruct, but merely utters 'beep', spells the patient's name and states the test name. DIVOTS may talk to, and receive data from, up to 15 stations simultaneously.

Within the laboratory Triage area, there is an automatic printer directly connected by hard-wire to the 370. It prints, pin-feed, fan-folded, sequentially numbered, pre-printed and pre-punched laboratory requisitions. At the start of each day, the laboratory clerk transmits to the 370, the number of the first available requisition. This specimen number is merged by the 370 with the hospital number of the 1st patient for whom tests are ordered. Henceforth, all subsequent, sequentially printed, requisitions will be merged automatically with the patients' hospital numbers as the tests are ordered.

Immediately after entry of an urgent test request, the 370 prints in the laboratory a requisition indicating the patient's name, age, sex, room, bed and hospital numbers and the tests desired. These data are entered on the human- and machine-readable punched stub-cards which will be attached to the specimen container for automatic identification (Fig. 4).

For non-urgent tests, the 370 will collect all orders for all patients of all wards as they are entered in random fashion. It will collate them by sequential ward, room and bed number and print patient requisitions every half hour in the same sequence and thus simplify specimen procurement for the phlebotomists.

In addition to printing the DIVOTS orders, the 370 transmits copies of these requests to the LDM to establish a list of anticipated test results. The 370 also bills the patient, counts the tests for statistical purposes and if a result is eventually not entered, it reminds the LDM later to satisfy the order or check on its absence.

The phlebotomist proceeds to the wards, rooms and patients printed on the requisitions. She reads the patient's name on the wrist-band, removes a pressure label and attaches it to the stubcard above the hospital number printed by the 370. They must be the same, thus verifying the accuracy of patient identification (Fig. 4).

When the phlebotomist returns to the laboratory with the specimens, they are 'logged in' by inserting the specimen stub-cards into the SPEC-IDENT®, a special specimen-identification device, thus maintaining a continuous 'audit trail' (Fig. 6). The tests are performed on multiple automated and semi-automated instruments and by manual methods. The stub-cards are used again in all systems for specimen identification. The results are processed by the LDM and transmitted to the 370 as described above to be filed in the patients' records.

Retrieval of test results by DIVOTS

To obtain results as early as possible, ward clerks and physicians initiate an essentially similar DIVOTS telephone transaction except that Codes 3 or 4 are used (3 for beginners and 4 for experienced clerks). After the hospital number is entered, the patient's name is spelled out audibly and thus verified. A special feature to guarantee the confidentiality of the test result at this point, is a program requirement to enter the attending physician's secret number to establish

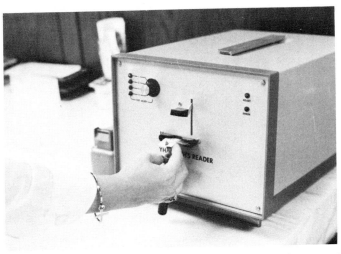

Fig. 6. The SPEC-IDENT® reads the pre-punched specimen number on the stub-card and merges it with the result in the LDM before transmission to the 370. It can also log in the sample arrival time in the laboratory.

his right to obtain the results on his patient. The computer will compare that number with the physician officially listed in the patient's record.

Test codes are then entered and audibly verified. One may inquire for any abnormal results only that day, all results for that day, or any result on any date during the patient's entire period of hospitalization. Single tests or entire organ or disease profiles are available. The audio-response system speaks the results sufficiently slowly to permit the hearer to write the message. A request to repeat the message may be accomplished by using the asterisk key.

Auto-call: DIVOTS automatic telephone dial-up

The 370 automatically dials the patient's nursing station telephone number as soon as it receives a special category of results from the LDM. This class consists of 'Stat' or urgently required results for seriously ill patients in Intensive or Coronary Care Units or, when abnormal results are obtained at any time, in tests of substances of potentially great medical hazard (i.e. potassium, blood sugar). When the phone is answered, the hearer is alerted by a chime, indicating a DIVOTS 'Auto-Call' message. The patient's name is spelled, the test is stated

```
                    DIVOTS ACTIVITY BY DOCTOR
          DOCTOR
    -------------------                                                    PAGE  12
BUTCHER G A MD                                  ORDERS              INQUIRIES
NUMBER              PATIENT        WARD   TEST NAME    TIME     TEST NAME    TIME
------              -------        ----   ---------    ----     ---------    ----
8143390     FAIRALL SALLY L        3NW   CBC        5  12/56/18
8133808     JENKINS JOSEPH         2NW   CBC        5  13/07/54
                                         PLATELET   5  13/07/54
8137927     WADE ELMER M           ICU   GROUP A    5  12/04/56
                                         CBC        5  12/04/56
                                         LDH        5  12/04/56
                                         S-GOT      5  12/04/56
                                         ENZ.-CPK   5  12/04/56
                                         LDH ISO.   5  12/04/56
8144567     BUCHANAN WILLIAM C     999                         PROT.ELECT   11/37/12
8143390     FAIRALL SALLY L        3NW   PCV        5  16/36/53
                                         HGB        5  16/36/53
                                         RETIC.     5  16/36/53
8133808     JENKINS JOSEPH         159                         CBC          16/54/22
8137927     WADE ELMER M           159                                      16/43/58
8139504     WALSH JOHN T           159                         LDH          16/51/31
```

Fig. 7. Portions of the S/7 daily log of DIVOTS usage. Note the listing by physician, the patients' test orders and results requested (inquiries) and the times of day of these transactions.

and the result is rendered. Thus, it is obvious that any delay between test result availability and its transmission to the physician is completely eliminated. We know of nothing as automatic or rapid for patient care as this process, which is completely independent of human effort.

Industrial engineering operations research and systems analysis are major components of our research on DIVOTS. Cost benefits of our audio-response communications system are being determined and compared with other conventional systems, printers and CRT's, and it has already been established conclusively that DIVOTS is far more economical. The telephone cost is practically negligible. Humans have no difficulty interfacing to the system since the familiar telephone poses no psychologic or intellectual hazards to nursing personnel.

DIVOTS' application already has expanded beyond the confines of the laboratory since we are now using it to discharge patients and are beginning to study its potential in the Pharmacy, starting with drug ordering and including inventory control. DIVOTS presents a daily log of all DIVOTS tests ordered and results requested. We are analyzing the physicians' reactions to the information (Fig. 7).

Conclusion

This is a brief description of the state of computer art in laboratory data acquisition, specimen identification, laboratory information and audio-response communications systems at the Youngstown Hospital Association and presents evidence of the potential technical possibilities inherent in such methodologies.

The impact of this technology on quality control test reliability and speed in all segments of the test cycle should be obvious to all experienced laboratory technicians. They include:

1. Elimination of errors in patient and test name identification because of DIVOTS audible verification.

2. Test result reliability is enhanced by eliminating the error-prone, man-pencil-paper interface.

3. Preparation of printed requisitions eliminates illegibility and faulty message interpretation.

4. Printing requisitions in the laboratory eliminates personnel delivery time and delay in initiating test performance. Transfer of pre-printed, hospital numbered labels from the patient's wrist-band to the human- and machine-readable stub-card verifies patient and sample identification.

5. Availability of test results immediately after test performance and prior to printing reports, assists physicians in early decision making and initiating appropriate treatment rapidly, thus improving patient care. Results are obtained

easily and reliably through any T-T telephone and expensive and cumbersome CRT's are not required.

6. Reduced length of hospitalization through earlier treatment cuts costs without sacrificing quality of patient care.

7. DIVOTS permits significant economies by reducing total labor costs on nursing stations and in the laboratory.

References

Keller, H. (1975): *Med. Lab., 28,* 1.

Lewis, H. L. (1975): *Mod. Healthcare, 3,* 16.

Rappoport, A. E. (Ed.) (1971): In: *IV International Symposium on Quality Control,* p. 114. Hans Huber, Berne.

Rappoport, A. E. (1973): In: *Laboratory Medicine,* Chapter 23, p. 1. Editor: G. J. Race. Harper and Row, New York.

Rappoport, A. E. and Gennaro, W. D. (1974): In: *Computers in Biomedical Research,* Chapter 4, p. 215. Editors: R. W. Stacy and B. D. Waxman. Academic Press, New York.

Rappoport, A. E., Gennaro, W. D. and Berquist, R. E. (1975a): In: *Proceedings, National Computer Conference, Anaheim, Calif.,* p. 757. Volume 44, AFIPS Press, Montvale, N.J.

Rappoport, A. E., Gennaro, W. D. and Constandse, W. J. (1967): *Mod. Hosp., 108,* 107.

Rappoport, A. E., Gennaro, W. D. and Constandse, W. J. (1968): *Mod. Hosp., 110,* 94.

Rappoport, A. E., Gennaro, W. D. and Berquist, R. E. (1975b): *Lab. Med., 6,* 22.

Rappoport, A. E. and Rappoport, E. (1970): *Hospitals, 44,* 114.

Rappoport, A. E., Constandse, W. J., Seligson, D. and Greanias, E. C. (Ed.) (1964): *Proceedings, Symposium on Computer-Assisted Pathology, Florida.* College of American Pathologists, Chicago.

8: Accuracy assessment and target values

K. G. von Boroviczény[1], A. von Klein-Wisenberg[2], R. Merten[3], U. P. Merten[4] and V. Schumann[3]

[1]Geschäftsstelle und Abteilung Methodologie, Berlin, [2]Abteilung Analytik und Numerik, Freiburg and [3]Abteilung Qualitätssicherung, Düsseldorf, Institut für Standardisierung und Dokumentation im Medizinischem Laboratorium (INSTAND), and [4]Institut für Virologie, University of Cologne, Federal Republic of Germany

Introduction

Presented by R. Merten

The Calibration Act which passed the German Parliament in 1969 introduced into laboratory medicine the legal compulsion to set up a scheme of internal quality control and to participate in external quality assessment comparative trials. Whereas internal laboratory quality control finds its main objective in the control chart, establishing the so-called 'true' value, or rather the 'assigned' value, presents the main problem. As we all know, not being omniscient, no true value can be defined, but only divined. The assessment of assigned or true values will be discussed from different aspects.

The model discussed in the first paper originates from and is an adaption of the ISCH standard procedure for the estimation of haemoglobin concentration on the international cyanmethaemoglobin standard, which was established as early as 1964 in Stockholm with the participation of members of our Institute and several other international experts.

This is the minimum which can be done for the assessment of target values and can easily be implemented, as shown in the following contributions dealing with the results from several reference laboratories. The question of the exact number of 'several' depends on many experimental circumstances and the probability limits considered suitable for the constituents in question. Apart from statistical reasons, it is common-sense experience that a target value gains plausibility when corroborated by many laboratories.

Practical experience with the procedures outlined has shown that – in regard to homogeneous analytical procedures – the target values found according to our scheme agreed fairly well with the mean of a large number of laboratories which can be considered to work under quality control and represent the present state of the art. On the other hand, discrepancies have been revealed, not only between different methods for the determination of a certain constituent, but also between reagent kits of different makes for the same method.

As long as there are no standard methods universally agreed upon, it is regrettably essential to evaluate comparative trials with these constituents separately, depending on the method and reagent kit used. This is clearly deplorable and highly uneconomic. It is hoped that the users and producers concerned will find a way in the near future to agree on standard methods. These need not yield the 'true' value, whatever we mean by that, but they should give reproducible and consistent results.

The papers presented here are the result of many discussions and experiments. No specific authorship can be attributed to any particular person concerned.

Highly accurate (assured) values in medical laboratories

Presented by K. G. von Boroviczény

From time to time, in all laboratories, it is necessary to evaluate a test with the best possible accuracy: (1) a test may be not accepted by the clinician if it does · not fit his clinical diagnosis; (2) the indication for an operation may depend on a single test result; (3) a test may establish a target value in a survey; (4) a test may establish a target value for reference material. These tests must be highly accurate and much work is required to obtain these 'assured' values. It is impossible to do this with all routine tests; since the work required is too great. The necessary work can be done in only a few cases with these special indications.

We would like to present a method for determining these 'assured' values. The method has been used for years for the evaluation of target values in the reference laboratories of the Institute for Standardization and Documentation in Medical Laboratories (INSTAND), and in other special cases in our hospital. The method can be used only in medium size or large laboratories; small laboratories should send their doubtful results to larger ones for confirmation.

Our method was devised to provide the most accurate results with a minimum of additional laboratory work. It requires 2 technicians familiar with the method and 2 separate, fully equipped working places in the laboratory. This includes dilutors, photometers, etc. It is desirable, but not essential, to have 2 different but compatible methods for the analyses, e.g. polarographic and photometric

TABLE 1

Cause of errors	Gross faults	Random errors	Systematic errors
Environment	+ x	(x)	(+) x
Apparatus	+ (x)	xx	xxx
Technicians	++ (x)	+ x	xx
Methods	+	xx	xx
Reagents	x	(x)	(+) x
Samples	+	x	+

+ = single analyses error.
x = series of errors.

glucose-oxidase reaction for blood glucose determinations, and manual and electronic blood-cell counting methods.

The theoretical background of our method is shown in Table 1. Gross errors can be avoided by careful work, and random errors can be adjusted and computed by making more than one test. It is of great importance to avoid systematic bias; so our method allows small systematic errors to be compensated for, and larger ones can at least be detected. Errors introduced by the environment can be detected by conducting the tests on 2 different days. Because of the nature of systematic apparatus errors and systematic personnel errors it is important that the 2 technicians work in separate places. Errors caused by the methods can be detected only when 2 different but comparable methods are used. To avoid systematic errors caused by the reagents, different batches of reagents should be used at the 2 working places, and the same applies when only one method is available. It may be advantageous to use reagents from 2 different companies.

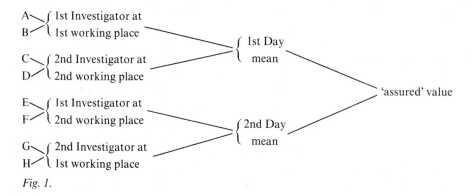

Fig. 1.

Errors caused by the sample itself can be avoided, or at least detected, if at least 4 separate vials are used in the tests.

Figure 1 shows an outline of the testing scheme. 2 technicians at 2 working places test the specimen on 2 days in duplicate. If all 8 values are available, the first thing to be considered is their dispersion: are they randomly distributed or is one value (or a pair) markedly different from the others (outliers)? One must also determine whether there is a relevant difference between the 2 working places, the 2 technologists, or the 2 days.

Tests for statistically significant differences can be made, but unless they are clinically relevant, small differences can be neglected. If the above questions can be answered satisfactorily, the mean value and the standard error of the mean can be computed. This is the 'assured' value.

Statistical models and confidence intervals in the assessment of target values

Presented by A. von Klein-Wisenberg

Hat von Euch jeder seinen Ring vom Vater: so glaube
jeder sich seinen Ring den echten.
(G. E. Lessing: *Nathan der Weise*, III, 7)

The problem posed by the assignment of 'true' values for quality control standard samples for clinical pathology is related to the famous ring parable quoted above: the father bequeathing to each of his three sons the purportedly real ring, with the subsequent confrontation of three legitimate owners of the real thing. We therefore much prefer to call the result of the assessment of the nominal value of a constituent in a quality control sample the 'target' or 'assigned' value.

The assessment of target values is usually effected by replicate analysis of the –allegedly homogeneous and uniformly distributed –sample in different laboratories using a specified method and stating the equipment being used. We assume for further evaluation, accepting the central limit theorem of mathematical statistics, that the scatter of the experimental results about the mean is normally distributed with homogeneous variance, so that parametric statistical tests can be applied. With only a limited number of laboratories available, tests for the validity of the first assumption –normal distribution –are not very significant and are usually omitted. The second assumption –homogeneity of variance –may be tested by performing multiple F-tests or Bartlett's test, provided the variance is not zero.

In simple determinations, when the uncertainty in instrument reading is the limiting factor of accuracy, e.g. haematocrit or haemoglobin determinations, or when instrument readings are converted by tables to the concentrations asked for, this may present a problem. To avoid zero variance in the laboratory, the participants are told to report replicate values with their inherent scatter; otherwise calculations must be made carrying one more than the least significant decimal, this being filled with uniformly distributed random numbers.

When the data of each laboratory agree with the hypothesis of equal variance, we may proceed further. If not, the records should be scrutinized for suspected outliers which are very probably responsible for this finding. Since we have assumed normal distribution, range tests such as Dixon's or Nalimov's may be applied to suspected outliers. The confidence limit of 95% has proved adequate for all tests. After outlying results in each laboratory have been excluded without substitution of the deleted value(s), comparison of variances is once more performed. If inequality is again found, the explanation will usually be methodological. Grossly scattered data from one or a few laboratories will lead to the exclusion of those data from further evaluation.

The consistent gross scatter within laboratories, numerically defined as the 'within-laboratory' variance of the unifactorial scheme of analysis, provides a measure for comparing different laboratory results by Scheffé's method of linear contrasts. This can lead to valuable findings: creatinine determinations by the method of Jaffé which were examined in this way showed significantly different results between the users of two different makes of reagent kit; the results of cholesterol determinations performed by the Liebermann-Burchardt method are considerably higher than those obtained by enzymatic determination.

From a clinical point of view these findings are of course deplorable, but the ascertainment of incompatible and uncomparable methods will hopefully lead to increasing standardisation on a world-wide scale, as has already been achieved with haemoglobinometry. For the present time the person or institution in charge of the assessment of target values must be aware of methodological differences in results and must state the different target values, if they can be ascertained. However, target values should not be given unless they are based on the results of at least 4 laboratories. This agrees with the draft of an ISO standard (ISO-TC 69/N 200): 'The determination of repeatability and reproducibility', where a figure of 8-15 laboratories is preferred. The impossibility of stating target values for seriously wrong or exotic methods will hopefully lead in the long run to increased comparability of results.

The confidence limit of the stated target value is estimated from the sum of variances within and between laboratories using the t-distribution, 95% two-sided probability, with 1 less than the total number of laboratories as the degree of freedom. There is still a long way to go to the goal of comparability. We have taken a few steps which have turned out to be promising, encouraging and challenging. It is to be hoped that communicative cooperation will lend impetus to the combined effort needed.

TECHNICAL NOTE 1: Considerations of different statistical models with their confidence intervals in the assessment of target values

The statistical method of analysis of variance is one of the most versatile tools in studying the many influences which may affect a measurement. The analysis of variance is itself part of the general linear model, in which a random variable y depends on p known quantities $x_1.....x_p$ and on p unknown parameters $b_1...b_p$.

$$y = b_1x_1 + b_2x_2 .... + b_px_p + e \tag{1}$$

where e (error) is a random variable with a mean of zero and a variance of σ^2.

In a simple case a specimen sample is given to p laboratories, each doing n measurements (replicates). The model now is:

$$y_{ij} = \mu + \alpha_i + \epsilon_{ij} \tag{2}$$

where i = laboratory index ($i = 1 .... p$),
            j = replicate index ($j = 1 .... n$),
            μ = general mean and
            α_i = effect of ith laboratory.

The hypothesis is: $\alpha_i = 0$ for all laboratories, which in the analysis of variance is tested by the F-test. If the test is positive, a suitable multiple comparison test (Scheffé or Tukey) can be done to see which laboratories differ significantly from the mean and should therefore perhaps be excluded from further consideration. Different methods may also influence the measurements, and to test for these we must enlarge our model:

$$y = \mu + \alpha_i + \beta_{ij} + e \tag{3}$$

Here α_i is the influence of each method, and β_{ij} is the influence of the jth laboratory for the ith method. Since it is unusual for a laboratory to perform all methods, we have to use different laboratories for each method. Thus the laboratories will be linked with the methods, and we have a nested design.

So far each influence has been considered to be fixed. But, for instance, in model (2) we often want to generalize to many laboratories, so that the influence α_i of the ith laboratory is of interest only in that it is considered as a random effect, since the laboratory may be taken to be a random sample from a whole population of laboratories. The total variance of a measurement y can now be separated into two components:

variance component for laboratories $= \sigma^2\alpha$

variance component for analytical precision $= \sigma^2 e$

A confidence limit for the general mean can be calculated as:

$$\bar{X} \pm t\,(1-2,p-1) \quad \sqrt{S_\alpha^2 + S_e^2} \tag{4}$$

In the fixed effects models there is only the estimate of the pure experimental error, and confidence intervals can be estimated easily when effects are not significant.

TECHNICAL NOTE 2: Determination of confidence limits based on analytical precision and clinical relevance in clinical chemistry with special regard to methods and clinical relevance

Clinical relevance in this context is taken to mean the maximum imprecision in a determination tolerable in relation to practical necessity. Tonk's criterion is a well known approach to the problem. A more recent proposal by the FDA suggests 8% of the normal range as a maximum measure of imprecision. In a concrete case such a relevant deviation can be expressed as a multiple of the standard deviation of the method used. If laboratory bias can be considered fixed (Technical note 1, model (2)), Table 1 and Figure 1 show the number of laboratories needed, when each supplies 4, 6 or 12 determinations, to detect those laboratories working outside the permissible relevant range with a discriminating power of 95%, when testing with a 5% level of significance.

Considerations of this kind, together with practical experience, have led IN-STAND to maintain that about 10 laboratories with 4 determinations each are ideal for most cases.

We will here give two examples, the determination of creatinine and of cholesterol, to show how to obtain a target value with the corresponding confidence interval. In this method laboratory effects are first regarded as fixed, so that multiple comparison methods may point out possible outliers. Laboratory effects are then considered in a random way in order to estimate variance components and confidence intervals for the means, which are then viewed as target values.

The values from 10 laboratories using the kinetic method for determining creatinine are shown in Table 2. The analysis of variance (Table 3) suggested discrepancies between the laboratories. Multiple comparisons between the means revealed a pattern, and two distinct groups can be recognized. It was then

TABLE 1

No. of deter-minations in each laboratory	Number of laboratories needed	Relevant imprecision as a multiple of the standard deviation
4	2	1.52
	4	1.21
	6	1.05
	8	0.94
	10	0.87
	12	0.82
	14	0.77
	16	0.71
	18	0.69
	20	0.67
6	2	1.13
	4	0.92
	6	0.80
	8	0.73
	10	0.67
	12	0.64
	14	0.60
	16	0.58
	18	0.56
	20	0.54
12	2	0.74
	4	0.61
	6	0.54
	8	0.49
	10	0.46
	12	0.43
	14	0.41
	16	0.39
	18	0.38
	20	0.37

Example: If each laboratory does 4 determinations, and a mean relevant imprecision of 0.82 standard deviation from the mean is tolerated for a laboratory, then at least 12 laboratories are needed to establish whether the common performance is within the permissible range.

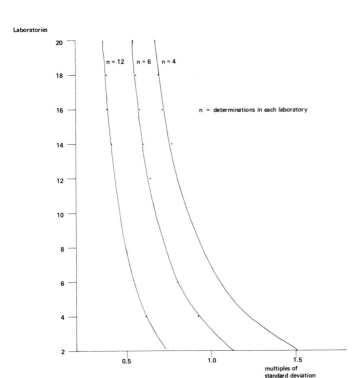

Fig. 1.

found that this grouping was due to two different reagent kits being used: one group had used mainly Boehringer reagent kits and the other Merck reagent kits. The analysis was therefore repeated for the two reagent groups and the

TABLE 2

Values (mg/dl) obtained by 10 laboratories using the kinetic method for determining creatinine

	1	2	3	4	5	6	7	8	9	10
	4.13	3.14	3.57	4.32	4.13	4.21	3.18	3.27	3.62	4.54
	4.27	3.30	3.67	4.21	4.08	4.24	3.28	3.15	3.50	4.45
Mean	4.20	3.22	3.62	4.26	4.10	4.22	3.23	3.21	3.56	4.49
Rank order	4	9	6	2	5	3	8	10	7	1

TABLE 3

Multiple comparisons between laboratory means (after Scheffé)

Reagent	Boehr	self-pre-pared	Roche	Boehringer		Merck				
Laboratory	10	4	6	1	5	3	9	7	2	8
Mean	4.49	4.26	4.22	4.20	4.10	3.62	3.56	3.23	3.22	3.21
4.26	0.23									
4.22	0.27	0.04								
4.20	0.29	0.06	0.02							
4.10	0.39	0.16	0.12	0.09						
3.62	0.87	0.64	0.60	0.58	0.48					
3.56	0.93	0.70	0.66	0.64	0.54	0.06				
3.23	1.26	1.03	0.99	0.97	0.87	0.39	0.33			
3.22	1.27	1.04	1.00	0.98	0.88	0.40	0.34	0.01		
3.21	1.28	1.05	1.01	0.99	0.89	0.41	0.35	0.02	0.01	

$K = \sqrt{9 \times 3.02 \times 0.0059} = 0.40$

TABLE 4

Results of analysis of variance in kinetic determinations of creatinine using two different reagent kits

	Boehringer	Merck
Laboratory variance component	0.0189	0.038
Method variance component	0.0043	0.007
Variance for the mean	0.0042	0.008
S.D.	0.065 (S% = 1.53)	0.091 (S% = 2.71)
Variance for a single value	0.0232	0.045
S.D.	0.152 (S% = 3.57)	0.213 (S% = 6.32)
Total mean (mg/dl)	4.26	3.37
95% confidence interval for the mean	4.08-4.44	3.12-3.62
95% confidence interval for a single value	3.84-4.68	2.78-3.96

TABLE 5

Values (mg/dl) obtained by 13 laboratories for creatinine using several end-point methods

	1	2	3	4	5	6	7	8	9	10	11	12	13
	4.05	4.33	4.62	4.07	4.53	4.86	3.97	4.14	3.78	4.15	3.92	4.11	4.05
	4.11	4.67	4.53	4.07	4.50	4.82	3.87	4.22	3.79	4.16	3.95	4.16	4.05
Mean	4.08	4.50	4.57	4.07	4.51	4.84	3.92	4.18	3.78	4.15	3.93	4.13	4.05
Rank order	8	4	2	9	3	1	12	5	13	6	11	7	10

results are shown in Table 4. Merck reagents yielded significantly lower values than Boehringer reagents, and seemed to be less precise.

Table 5 shows the results when creatinine was determined using several end-point methods. Although significant discrepancies between laboratory means were found, the cause could not be determined. The results are shown in Tables 6 and 7.

TABLE 6

Multiple comparisons between laboratory means (after Scheffé)

Laboratory	6	3	5	2	8	10	12	1	4	13	11	7	9
Method	TCA	AA	TCA	AA	PA	TCA	PA	TCA	AA	PA	TCA	AA	TCA
Mean	4.84	4.58	4.52	4.50	4.18	4.16	4.13	4.08	4.07	4.05	3.94	3.92	3.79
4.58	0.26												
4.52	0.32	0.06											
4.50	0.34	0.08	0.02										
4.18	0.66	0.40	0.34	0.32									
4.16	0.68	0.42	0.36	0.34	0.02								
4.13	0.71	0.45	0.39	0.37	0.05	0.03							
4.08	0.76	0.50	0.44	0.42	0.10	0.08	0.05						
4.07	0.77	0.51	0.45	0.43	0.11	0.09	0.06	0.01					
4.05	0.79	0.53	0.47	0.45	0.13	0.11	0.08	0.03	0.02				
3.94	0.90	0.64	0.58	0.56	0.24	0.22	0.19	0.14	0.13	0.11			
3.92	0.92	0.66	0.60	0.58	0.26	0.24	0.21	0.21	0.16	0.15	0.13	0.02	
3.79	1.05	0.79	0.73	0.71	0.39	0.37	0.34	0.29	0.28	0.28	0.26	0.15	0.13

$K = \sqrt{12 \times 2.60 \times 0.0058} = 0.43$
TCA = trichloracetic acid, AA = autoanalyzer, PA = picric acid.

TABLE 7

Analysis of variance in creatinine determinations by end-point methods

Laboratory variance component	0.090
Method variance component	0.006
Variance for the mean	0.007
S.D.	0.085 (S% = 2.51)
Variance for a single value	0.096
S.D.	0.310 (S% = 7.37)
Total mean (mg/dl)	4.21
95% confidence interval for the mean	4.03-4.40
95% confidence interval for a single value	3.54-4.89

TABLE 8

Values (mg/dl) obtained by 8 laboratories for cholesterol using the enzymatic method

	1	2	3	4	5	6	7	8
	141.0	152.3	152.0	133.0	138.3	151.3	152.0	135.0
	133.0	147.7	155.0	136.7	138.7	139.3	150.0	138.0
Mean	137.0	150.0	153.5	134.8	138.5	145.3	151.0	136.5
Rank order	6	3	1	8	5	4	2	7

Analysis of variance

Laboratory variance component	47.81
Method variance component	16.56
Variance for the mean	7.01
S.D.	2.65 (S% = 1.85)
Variance for a single value	64.37
S.D.	8.02 (S% = 5.60)
Total mean (mg/dl)	143.3
95% confidence interval for the mean	137.1-149.6
95% confidence interval for a single value	124.3-162.3

TABLE 9

Values (mg/dl) obtained by 10 laboratories for cholesterol using the Liebermann-Burchardt method

	1	2	3	4	5	6	7	8	9	10
	148.7	146.7	160.3	166.3	164.3	161.0	165.3	169.0	173.0	173.0
	153.3	145.0	156.7	161.0	161.7	190.7	158.0	180.3	169.7	170.3
Mean	151.0	145.8	158.5	163.6	163.0	175.8	161.6	174.6	171.3	171.6
Rank order	9	10	8	5	6	1	7	2	4	3

Analysis of variance

Laboratory variance component	71.27
Method variance component	57.66
Variance for the mean	10.01
S.D.	3.16 (S% = 1.93)
Variance for a single value	128.93
S.D.	11.35 (S% = 6.93)
Total mean	163.7
95% confidence interval for the mean	156.6-170.8
95% confidence interval for a single value	138.0-189.4

These results show that the kinetic method using Boehringer reagents compared well with other end-point methods, but that the kinetic method using Merck reagents yielded significantly lower results in this case.

In Tables 8 and 9 the determination of cholesterol by the enzymatic method is compared with that by the Liebermann-Burchardt method. The results have been analysed in the same way as in the creatinine example. The enzymatic method yielded significantly lower values than the Liebermann-Burchardt method, so that individual target values must be given for both methods.

Target values for evaluating results in collaborative surveys

Presented for R. Merten by U. P. Merten

It has been shown that the number of laboratories needed for obtaining a target value can be estimated on the basis of statistical models, provided that some assumptions about precision and accuracy are agreed upon. There is an FDA proposal to use 8% of the normal range as a measure of accuracy, but this seems to be difficult in practice. Table 1 shows a comparison for selected substances between this measure of accuracy and that found for some target value determinations by INSTAND. For the INSTAND results the measure was defined as 4 times the standard error of the mean.

A further possibility would be to use the relative empirical standard deviations, as previously found, or perhaps some suitable multiples of the relative standard deviation, to set up a tolerance interval for a determination. However, this still leaves the problem that estimates vary according to the different investigators and the methods, reagent kits and concentration levels used.

Formerly we used the 2S interval around a target value as the tolerance interval; this was done individually for each specimen. In Tables 2, 3, 4 and 5 average relative standard deviations from 1972 to 1974 for all common constituents are shown. These averages reflect the measuring abilities of specialist laboratories, and could also be used to establish tolerance intervals. Our calculations have shown that 95% of the determinations done by reference laboratories for different constituents can be roughly classified into 5 groups: (1) $\bar{x} \pm 5\%$; (2) $\bar{x} \pm$

TABLE 1

Required accuracy ranges (tolerance) for target values

Substance	Standard	Normal range*	Differ-ence	Measure of accuracy	Target value examples from reference laboratories				
					x̄	S%	S	S x̄	n (ref. lab.)
Chloride (mmol/l)	FDA	98 to 110	12	1.0	102.2	2.3	2.35	0.6	16
mercurimetric	INSTAND			2.4	102.3	2.3	2.35	0.6	16
colorimetric	INSTAND			2.0			2.06	0.5	16
Sodium (mmol/l)	FDA	135 to 150	15	1.2					
	INSTAND			3.6	142.5	2.43	3.46	0.9	16
Glucose (mg/dl)	FDA	60 to 100	40	3.2					
	INSTAND			6.7	123.2	4.06	5.0	1.67	9
Uric acid (mg/dl)	FDA	3.5 to 6.5	3.0	0.24					
	INSTAND			0.20	4.67	4.46	0.21	0.05	17
Urea (mg/dl)	FDA	8.5 to 39.2	30.7	2.5					
	INSTAND			2.0	39.5	4.87	1.92	0.5	16

* See W. Rick (1974): In: *Clinical Chemistry and Microscopy, 3rd ed.,* pp. 391 ff. Springer, Berlin.

TABLE 2

Average relative standard deviations (S%) for the period 1972 to 1974 for inorganic substances

Substance	Concentration range		Units	No. of determinations	S%
	from	to			
Calcium	1.75	3.22 ⎫	mmol/l	1725	4.24
Chloride	84	115 ⎭		1698	2.48
Copper	13.8	25.3 ⎫	μmol/dl	975	6.79
Iron	11.3	36.7 ⎭		976	6.57
Lithium	0.86	5.48 ⎫		551	4.16
Magnesium	0.66	2.30 ⎪		1111	6.15
Phosphorus, inorg.	1.1	2.65 ⎬	mmol/l	795	5.76
Potassium	3.5	7.6 ⎪		1606	3.77
Sodium	100	145 ⎭		1545	2.08

TABLE 3

Average relative standard deviations (S%) for the period 1972 to 1974 for organic substances

Substance	Concentration range (mg/dl)		No. of determinations	S%
	from	to		
Bilirubin	0.4	5.5	1414	6.37
Cholesterol	117	189	1259	5.95
Creatinine	1.0	4.7	1129	5.92
Glucose	82	268	1801	4.54
Lipids (total)	434	709	246	6.48
Protein (total)	5.1	8.2	1539	3.40
Triglycerides	38	116	462	6.22
Urea	20	117	1596	5.66
Uric Acid	3.2	10.0	1428	5.50

TABLE 4

Average relative standard deviations (S%) for the period 1972 to 1974 for enzymes

Substance	Concentration range (U/l)		No. of determinations	S%
	from	to		
AP, not optimized	30	128	300	11.3
AP, optimized	47	263	419	8.87
CK, activated	8	190	514	10.3
γ-GT	12	71	1062	7.66
GOT, not optimized	14	65	593	7.26
GOT, optimized	16	130	398	7.51
GPT, not optimized	4	102	599	9.56
GPT, optimized	5	286	381	11.1
LAP	8	63	439	10.6
LDH	112	1240	554	8.91
LDH-1-Isoenzyme	82	279	427	7.44
SP (total)	7.1	62.3	461	9.70
PSP	0.85	55.7	438	10.76

AP = alkaline phosphatase, CK = creatine kinase, γ-GT = glutamyltranspeptidase, GOT = glutamic-oxaloacetic transaminase, GPT = glutamic-pyruvic transaminase, LAP = leucyl-arylamidase, LDH = lactate dehydrogenase, SP = acid phosphatase, PSP = prostatic acid phosphatase.

TABLE 5

Average relative standard deviations (S%) for the period 1972 to 1974 for concentrations in the normal and elevated range

Substance	Units	Upper normal limit	Concentration below upper normal limit		Concentration above upper normal limit	
			No.	S%	No.	S%
Bilirubin		1.0	224	6.90	1190	6.27
Glucose		110	836	4.93	965	4.16
Uric Acid	mg/dl	7.0	437	5.92	991	5.31
Urea		50	614	6.83	982	5.44
Creatinine		1.5	215	6.58	914	5.75
AP		200	476	10.70	243	8.24
CK		30	211	10.94	303	9.78
GOT, not optimized		20	140	7.33	453	7.24
GOT, optimized		20	70	11.59	328	6.30
GPT, not optimized		20	256	10.93	343	8.40
GPT, optimized	U/l	20	132	14.66	249	8.53
γ-GT		20	188	10.36	874	6.95
LAP		20	317	10.70	122	10.41
LDH		150	156	10.26	398	8.31
LDH-1-Isoenzyme		150	115	9.68	312	6.40
SP (total)		10	76	15.18	385	8.20
PSP		1	47	13.96	391	10.32

10%; (3) $\bar{x} \pm 15\%$; (4) (enzymes) $\bar{x} \pm 20\%$; (5) more than $\bar{x} \pm 20\%$ (enzymes). These groups are shown in Table 6 for selected substances.

It is also necessary to examine how accuracy is affected by different concentration levels. Tables 6 and 7 show this effect, which results in smaller relative standard deviations for higher concentrations, so that a decision at the clinically critical level is facilitated for most constituents.

It has already been proved that relative precision decreases at lower concentration levels. As a consequence of this well known fact, together with our findings, we decided to use only those control specimens in which all the constituents had concentrations about the upper clinical decision level. This was also recommended to the manufacturers of control specimens.

Strictly speaking, there are no adequate measures to ensure that the target value obtained represents the true value; since in biological material the true value cannot be determined, except for some inorganic constituents. There have been attempts to obtain values under comparable conditions, but it was found

TABLE 6

Classification of chemical constituents on the basis of empirical relative standard deviations and concentration levels below or above the upper normal limit

Concentration		Concentration		Concentration		Concentration		Concentration
below	above	below	above	below	above	below	above	above
S%<2.5		S%=2.5 to 5.0		S%=5.0 to 7.5		S%=7.5 to 10.0		S%>10.0
	Calcium	Calcium						
Chloride	Chloride		Lithium					
Sodium	Sodium			Magnesium	Magnesium	AP		AP
	Potassium	Potassium				CK		CK
			Phosporus	Phosphorus		GPT		GPT
		Glucose	Glucose	Bilirubin	Bilirubin	LDH		LDH
				Uric acid	Uric acid	SP		SP
				Urea	Urea			PSP
				Creatinine	Creatinine			
					GOT	GOT		
					γ-GT	γ-GT		

that the enormous effort and costs required were prohibitive for practical clinical purposes.

When confirming a target value in collaborative surveys we use the following procedures:

1. The target value is compared to the mean value from a selected group of laboratories, which are assumed to work satisfactorily.

2. The target value is compared to the mean value of all participants, after elimination of outliers.

3. If Step 1 shows differences, the means of the values of the reference laboratories will be weighted by a function of the variances, so that values from laboratories with excessively small or large variances will be multiplied or divided by a suitable factor.

These procedures have proved satisfactory in practice, so that deviation in means occurs only rarely, except for some enzymes. Participants in surveys often ask to be allowed to use the total mean instead of a target value established beforehand. There should perhaps be a discussion on which constituents such a procedure could be applied to and under what conditions.

Unfortunately there are diverse methods for the determination of a constituent. When methods show significant differences, they have to be taken into

TABLE 7

Methodological differences in target values

No difference		Noticeable differences between methods	
Inorganic			
Chloride	Calcium	Flame emission/atomic adsorption	Colour test: chloranilate precipitation
Lithium	Magnesium	Atomic adsorption	Colour test: xylidyl blue
Potassium	Phosphorus, inorg.	Colour test as phospho-molybdate blue without protein precipitation	Colour test: after protein precipitation; with ammonium molybdate vanadate or malachite green
Sodium			
Copper	Iron	Colour test: batho-phenanthroline without protein precipitation	Colour test: bathophenanthroline after protein precipitation; tripyridyl-triazine
Organic			
Bilirubin	Cholesterol	Colour test: after reaction with acetic anhydride, sulphuric acid (Liebermann/Burchardt)	Enzymatic colour test with cholesterol esterase/oxidase
	Glucose	Colour test after reaction with hexokinase/G-6-PDH	Colour test after reaction with GOD/ABTS (Perid®)
	Uric Acid	Colour test after oxidation with phosphotungstic acid	Enzymatic colour test after reaction with uricase/katalase; endpoint registration/continuous registration
	Urea	Urease cleavage and determination of ammonium (Berthelot)	Colour test after reaction with diacetyl monoxime
	Creatinine	Jaffé test with protein precipitation due to picric acid/tungstic acid/TCA	Jaffé test with continual (kinetic) registration
Enzymes			
	AP, CK, GLDH, GOT, GPT, LDH, LDH-1-Isoenzyme	Conventional 'non-optimized' methods	German standard methods with 'optimized concentrations' of substrates and co-enzymes at 25°C

TABLE 8

Comparison of target values with participant values

1st survey (1975)	Sample								
	Target value from reference laboratories			Selected group of participants			All participants		
	No.	x̄	S%	No.	x̄	S%	No.	x̄	S%
Sodium	33	135.20	2.43	15	134.90	2.85	194	134.90	8.36
Potassium	32	3.98	4.35	54	4.03	5.50	208	3.99	16.6
Calcium	30	2.13	2.62	53	2.14	5.89	218	2.16	21.1
Chloride	32	102.20	2.30	47	102.20	2.74	137	102.50	6.25
Phosphorus	18	1.16	4.2	33	1.15	7.63	128	1.20	36.5
Magnesium	32	0.95	4.34	26	0.96	9.38	59	0.93	37.7
Iron	18	21.00	6.33	14	20.90	7.22	65	23.50	63.3
Copper	15	21.90	4.57	31	23.70	11.00	82	23.30	31.8
Lithium	25	0.15	6.25				55	0.18	64.0

account when evaluating results from participants in surveys (see Table 7). Different reagent kits may also vary significantly with the same method, but further differentiation is certainty impractical (e.g. creatinine). Such discrepancies should be cleared up and eliminated.

At present our procedure for determining target values with tolerance intervals is as described in this paper.

Table 8 shows that differences in means between reference laboratories and a selected group of expert laboratories occur only rarely. On the other hand, there are sometimes differences between the target values and the means of all participants, which could be an argument for not taking the total mean as the target value.

Descriptors in clinical pathology

Presented by U. P. Merten

A large number of analytical results are returned to the evaluation centre when target values are established, and these results must be processed in a computer. In this processing not only the numerical results and their dimensions are important for accurate evaluation but also name of the test and the method applied.

For the calculation of target values as well as for general laboratory use, abbreviations are necessary for requests, storage, processing and reports of laboratory tests. The meaning of an abbreviation must be clear and its structure should not give rise to misunderstanding or confusion.

Abbreviations are usually composed by the laboratory itself, based on abbreviations found in the medical literature and in dictionaries. The result is that each laboratory specialty, such as chemistry, haematology, immunology or microbiology, has created its own vocabulary of abbreviations, and often the same abbreviation is used for different tests. For instance, capital 'C' has more than 40 meanings; 'TP' has at least 8, and 'LAP' has at least 3 (Schertel, 1974).

In future, a laboratory information system will have to cover all subspecialties in the clinical pathology laboratory and so all abbreviations have to be checked to avoid duplications. Some suggestions for the basic structure of laboratory abbreviations are presented in this paper. The idea is to combine different single abbreviations to create a 'descriptor', identifying not only the test itself, but also

TABLE 1

Abbreviations for laboratory units

B	Blood bank
C	Chemistry
E	Endocrinology
F	Fungi/Mycology
G	Genetics/Cytogenetics
H	Haematology
I	Immunology
M	Microbiology
N	Nuclear Medicine
P	Parasitology
S	Serology
T	Toxicology
V	Virology

the applied or requested method, the necessary or used specimen and the laboratory unit responsible.

Clinical pathology is subdivided into different subspecialties and the laboratory into different functional units. The description of each functional unit can be abbreviated with one capital letter, as shown in Table 1, and this letter indicates the responsible unit, which receives the specimen and working list and reports the results of quality controls and tests.

Depending on the test requested, a certain kind of specimen may be required and, vice versa, a given specimen sometimes requires a certain method to be used. For coagulation studies, for instance, primary plasma is needed, whereas serum and not plasma is used for complement-fixation tests. If an oral swab or stool is sent to the laboratory, isolation of a virus can be attempted but no complement-fixation test or neutralization test can be performed with these specimens.

The introduction of an abbreviation of up to 3 letters to indicate the nature of a specimen would make it possible to program for rejection if the specimen and the request did not fit. Some abbreviations for different specimens are listed in Table 2.

A computer can use the abbreviations of laboratory units and specimens to request a certain quality and/or quantity of specimen, or it can ask for division of the specimen sent in so that it is equally distributed to different laboratory units.

The kind of specimen required depends on the method applied, as does the 'normal' range. Therefore test, kind of specimen, method applied and normal

TABLE 2

Abbreviations for specimens

BFL	Blister fluid
BBS	Blister basal scraping
B	Blood
BW	Bronchial washing
CSF	Cerebrospinal fluid
CES	Cervical smear
F	Faeces
N	Nasal secretion
OS	Oral swab
PL	Plasma
S	Serum
SP	Sputum
SAL	Saliva
SK	Skin
THS	Throat swab
U	Urine

range should be treated as a unit, and in a computer program the abbreviations should be related to each other.

For abbreviations of tests, 6 to 8 letters seem to be sufficient and for methods 3. Some combinations of tests and methods are listed in Table 3.

We are trying to establish abbreviations covering English and German and as far as possible the Latin languages and French. It is difficult to prepare a catalogue listing all the different abbreviations of tests performed in clinical pathology laboratories and at the same time covering all the test names in more than two languages.

As a reference the internationally recognized table of chemical elements could be used. But even here problems arise, since many computers print capital letters only. Since most symbols of chemical elements represent quite short names,

TABLE 3

Some descriptors of test-method combination

FLU	–CFT	Influenza–Complement–fixation test
FLU	–HIT	Influenza–Haemagglutination inhibition test
FLU	–ISO	Influenza–Isolation
FERRUM–CEM		Iron–Chemical analysis
FERRUM–RIA		Iron–Radioimmunoassay

TABLE 4

Some descriptors in virology

V – BFL – VIRUS	– ISO	Blister fluid – Virus isolation
V – BFL – POX	– EM	Blister fluid – Poxvirus verification by electron microscopy
V – BFL – POX	– ISO	Blister fluid – Poxvirus isolation
V – S – CMV	– CFT	Serum – Cytomegalovirus – Complement-fixation test
V – S – CMV	– IGM	Serum – Cytomegalovirus – IGM
V – CES – CMV	– ISO	Cervical smear – Cytomegalovirus – Isolation
V – S – RUBEL	– HIT	Serum – Rubella – Haemagglutination inhibition test
V – S – RUBEL	– IGM	Serum – Rubella – IGM
V – THS – RUBEL	– ISO	Throat swab – Rubella – Isolation
V – F – ENTERO	– ISO	Faeces – Enterovirus – Isolation
V – S – ADENO	– CFT	Serum – Adenovirus – Complement-fixation test

these could be used in full in capital letters except when too long, or when integrated in an abbreviation of a chemical compound.

In addition, the International Code of Nomenclature of Bacteria is a valuable reference because the language problem is avoided. Other international commissions have established such classifications as SNOP and SNOMED related to the field of clinical pathology and these should be integrated into the fundamentals of clinical pathology descriptors. As an example some preliminary descriptors in virology are listed in Table 4.

It is evident that the length of such descriptors causes difficulties in recognizing their meaning and even a systematic grouping cannot really solve this problem.

A physician requesting a test from the laboratory seldom asks for a special method to be used in the test. He wants to know the proper test name and the kind of specimen required by the laboratory. Therefore the descriptor in virology, for instance, could be:

FLU or FLUA or FLUB.

But the physician should be able to request either a complement-fixation test or a haemagglutination inhibition test like this:

FLU –CFT or FLUA –CFT or FLUB –CFT
FLU –HIT or FLUA –HIT or FLUB –HIT.

Most often he will use the first form. The printout by the computer will list:

      V–S   –FLUA   –CFT

or V–S   –FLUB   –CFT

or the appropriate symbols for the HIT.

In clinical chemistry the physician should be able to request for instance:

      FERRUM

or FERRUM–CEM

or FERRUM–RIA

if the laboratory performs both methods. The computer printout will be either:

      C–S   –FERRUM–CEM

or C–S   –FERRUM–RIA.

The use of alphabetical-numerical symbols results in long descriptors which are primarily important for the identification of the laboratory's work. A physician asks for short symbols when requesting a test, especially when done by touch-tone telephone as at Dr. Rappoport's laboratory in Youngstown, Ohio, U.S.A. (see *This Volume*).

A numerical code seems to satisfy this purpose best. With 3 digits one can request and store up to 999 tests, combined with method, specimen, laboratory unit and 'normal' range, and we are all familiar with the use of telephone numbers. Every test name can be easily translated into a number without any language problem, but a dictionary is needed for requesting tests. Nevertheless the result will be reported with an abbreviated test name. Therefore codes for requests and abbreviations for reports have to be established. A disadvantage of numerical codes is the fixed combination of specimen, test and method, whereas a variable combination can be achieved with the alphabetical-numerical combination system explained above.

There are many pros and cons to both sides. The advantage of the alphabetical-numerical system is that it can be equally well used for requests, laboratory work and reports. If an international committee set up a catalogue with such descriptors covering the different languages, they could be used in the medical literature and in patient reports all over the world.

Reference

Schertel, A. (1974): *Abbreviations in Medicine*. S. Karger, Munich.

9: Standards in anatomic pathology

Standardization of nomenclature in anatomic pathology

R. A. Côté

Department of Pathology, Faculty of Medicine,
University of Sherbrooke, Sherbrooke, Quebec, Canada

The Commission on World Standards for Anatomic Pathology was established by the World Association of Societies of Pathology in an attempt to standardize various aspects of the practice of anatomic pathology. The first step towards this worthwhile goal must be the standardization of the nomenclature of pathology so that comparisons can be just and meaningful from one part of the world to the other.

In 1965, the College of American Pathologists published the 'Systematized Nomenclature of Pathology' (SNOP) mainly to code surgical and autopsy diagnoses. This was the result of about five years of cogitation on the part of one committee of the College of American Pathologists, the Committee on Nomenclature and Classification of Disease. Under the able leadership of its chairman, Doctor Arthur Wells, the final product represented a totally new approach to the coding of medical diagnoses in a four axis system.

Within a few years SNOP was translated into French, German, Japanese and other languages. From SNOP, the American Cancer Society prepared the 'Manual of Tumor Nomenclature and Coding' (MOTNAC) which was also translated into many more languages and has become the best available tool for tumor coding. This particular part of the morphology axis of SNOP has been recently revised by a committee of the World Health Organization and will soon be published as a separate fascicle called 'International Classification of Diseases for Oncology' (I.C.D.-O.).

For those who are still unfamiliar with SNOP, I will briefly outline the nomenclature.

All terms in SNOP are divided into four categories: topography, which is normal anatomy or structure; morphology, which is pathologic anatomy or structure; etiology, representing all agents capable of causing disease; and function, which is mostly a list of functional abnormalities and complex diseases as encountered by the pathologist. Whether knowingly or unknowingly, the pathologists had finally developed a true, although partial, basic medical nomenclature.

If SNOP was such a world-wide success in such a short time why are we now proposing SNOMED, a 'Systematized Nomenclature of Medicine'?

Concurrently with the acceptance of SNOP, investigators in medical computer sciences were still wrestling with the problem of the computerization of the medical record. It became gradually apparent that, to permit easy compact storage, and transfer and linkage of information, a basic systematized nomenclature of medicine was necessary. This same nomenclature must permit the coding of problems, signs, symptoms, disease entities, administrative, diagnostic and therapeutic procedures, all within the same framework. Realizing the need for such a framework, project directors began developing individual and mostly partial coding systems based on their own nomenclature. None encompassed the entire field of medicine.

Three years ago, following the expression of this national need, the Committee on Nomenclature and Classification of Disease of the College of American Pathologists, in collaboration with representatives of specialty societies, began developing a systematized nomenclature of medicine. This nomenclature will be divided into the following basic categories: topography, morphology, etiology, function, procedure and disease. It is the first attempt by modern medicine at developing a systematized nomenclature divided into specific categories which are philosophically sound.

This is an extension of SNOP to include two additional categories or axes. The old SNOP Function category was purified and complex disease entities and syndromes, both eponymic and non-eponymic, were organized into groups making up a separate category called 'Disease'. This is the category that actually represents multiples of the other nomenclature categories and can actually be considered as the classification component of the entire system.

To clarify this point take the example of tuberculosis. This is a complex entity

TABLE 1

Topography: numerical index

Section 0:	Integumentary, hematopoietic and lymphatic systems
Section 1:	Musculoskeletal and soft tissue systems
Section 2:	Respiratory tract
Sections 3 and 4:	Cardiovascular system
Sections 5 and 6:	Digestive system
Sections 7 and 8:	Genitourinary tract and fetal structures
Section 9:	Endocrine glands
Section X:	Nervous system and special sense organs
Section Y:	Topographic regions

TABLE 2

Morphology: numerical index

Section 0:	General nonspecific morphology
Section 1:	Traumatic abnormality
Section 2:	Developmental malformation
Section 3:	Mechanical abnormality
Section 4:	Inflammation and fibrosis
Section 5:	Degeneration, necrosis, deposition, dystrophy and atrophy
Section 6:	Macromolecular, chromosomal, and cytologic alteration
Section 7:	Growth and maturation alteration
Sections 8 and 9:	Neoplasm

TABLE 3

Etiology: numerical index

Section 0:	Etiology: general
Section 1:	Bacteria
Section 2:	Bacteria and Rickettsiae
Section 3:	Viruses
Section 4:	Other pathogenic organisms
Sections 5 and 6:	Chemicals – chemical elements
Sections 7 and 8:	Drugs and biologicals
Section 9:	Physical agents and therapeutic devices

TABLE 4

Function: numerical index

Section 0:	Functions and dysfunctional states of growth, growth periods and death
Sections 1 and 2:	Metabolic and endocrine functional units and states
Section 4:	Hematologic and immunologic functional units and states
Section 6:	Functions, functional states and abnormal functions of the digestive and urinary tracts
Section 7:	Functions, functional states and abnormal functions of the cardiovascular and respiratory systems
Section 8:	Functions, functional states and abnormal functions of the neuromuscular and skeletal systems
Section 9:	The psyche and the sexual state with normal and abnormal functions
Section X:	Functions and functional abnormalities of the eye and ear
Section Y:	Environmental circumstances surrounding physical injury or death

TABLE 5

Procedure: numerical index

Section 0:	General procedures
Section 1:	Operations and anesthesia
Sections 2, 3 and 4:	Systems-oriented special procedures
Section 5:	Radiography, radiation therapy, nuclear medicine and ultrasonic procedures
Sections 6, 7, 8 and 9:	Laboratory procedures
Section X:	Dental, oral and nursing procedures
Section Y:	Diets and home care procedures

in the Disease category which can be found in many different anatomic sites. The morphological expressions of the disease vary according to its stage and the functional expressions are many, from low grade fever, malaise, night sweats, cough and many more. Furthermore, the etiologic agent may be one or more different species or types of mycobacteria.

For recording diseases in general for statistical purposes, the Disease category or classification is sufficient. This is the portion that would serve the same purpose as the International Classification of Diseases, but for recording more specifically the separate components or manifestations of disease or its causative agents, the other categories of the nomenclature are essential.

TABLE 6

Disease: numerical index

Section 0:	Infectious and communicable diseases
Sections 1 and 2:	Metabolic and endocrine diseases and syndromes
Section 3:	Complex diseases and syndromes of the skeletal system, skin and connective tissues
Section 4:	Complex disorders, syndromes and diseases of the hematopoietic and immune systems
Section 6:	Diseases and syndromes of the digestive and urinary tracts
Section 7:	Diseases and syndromes of the cardiovascular and respiratory systems
Section 8:	Diseases and syndromes of the nervous and muscular systems
Section 9:	Emotional, mental and sexual diseases and syndromes
Section X:	Complex diseases and syndromes of the eye and ear

TABLE 7

Classification of amebiasis

	Nomenclature				
T	M	E	F	P	Classification
			Fever diarrhea		Disease-0016
Stools				Culture	Called
		E. histolytica			
		E. hartmanni			A
		(small forms)			M
Mucosa				Endoscopic	E
Colon				biopsy	B
Mucosa	Ulcerations	Ameba			I
Colon		(Trophozoites)			A
Liver				Series	S
Lung					I
Diaphragm	Abscess	Ameba		of	S
Kidney					
Stomach					
Duodenum				diagnostic	
Meninges					
Brain				procedures	006.0 ⎤
					006.1 ⎬ I.C.D.
					006.9 ⎦

The last category of the nomenclature is not directly concerned with the diagnostic statement, but is the action category and is called 'Procedure'. This is a list of administrative, diagnostic and therapeutic procedures necessary to make diagnoses and then to treat the patient.

The overall system for the total management of medical information is now complete. Anatomic and clinical pathology is now part of a broader concept embracing all aspects and all specialties of medicine. The SNOP philosophy of hierarchical categorization and coding has been extended with the help of our clinical colleagues and hopefully SNOMED will be the beginning of some standardization of the medical nomenclature in all languages.

Tables 1-6 show the one-digit content outline of each of the six categories. Using the elements from the six categories, one can code all the components of disease, including the procedures done at various levels in the diagnostic hierarchy. Table 7 shows components of the disease amebiasis which can be coded for statistical compilation as D-0016 or, in the International Classification of Diseases, as 006.0. The advantage of SNOMED is that all the various topographic sites can be coded separately as well as the different morphologic alterations seen by the pathologist. The proper etiologic agent as found by the microbiologist can also be specifically coded. Furthermore, the clinician can code all signs, symptoms and functional disturbances as well as the procedures done to diagnose and treat the disease. The SNOP system, expanded to SNOMED, is the only comprehensive medical data management tool now available.

The objectives of the Commission on World Standards for Anatomic Pathology are certainly to promote some form of standardization in pathology. Our aim is to promote the use of the time-tested SNOP and its successor, SNOMED. For those pathology groups or departments that are not yet using SNOP, we suggest that they begin early in 1976 with SNOMED. For those who are using SNOP, we feel that they could gradually make the change-over, after consultation with the Committee members. In summary, pathologists throughout the world, by beginning some form of standardization among themselves, will once again, by their foresight, example and dedication, lead the way for their colleagues in developing the tool that will serve the advancement of medicine as a science.

The pursuit of excellence in Australian surgical pathology

P. W. Allen

*Histopathology Division,
Institute of Medical and Veterinary Science, Adelaide, Australia*

The phrase, 'pursuit of excellence', was included in the title of this paper to suggest a laudable and even impressive undertaking; in practice, its real meaning should have been indiscernible. As far as I knew, it was an entirely original euphemism for examination of pathologists' diagnostic skills. After submitting this title to the conference organisers, I discovered that the College of American Pathologists used the same words on the front page of a booklet advertising its 'quality assurance programme', and, at this very meeting, there is a paper by Dr. J. D. Barger of Las Vegas entitled 'Laboratory excellence (inspection and accreditation)'. It seems that in the United States as well as in Australia the pleasant sound of 'excellence' is synonymous with the testing of pathologists' proficiency.

Pathologists in Australia have been concerned with their own excellence and status for many years, and although they were less than 200 strong, they banded together in 1956 and formed the College of Pathologists of Australia. The most important of its avowed 'missions' were:

1. 'To promote the study of the sciences and practice of pathology in relation to medicine; to encourage research in pathology and ancillary sciences; to bring

together pathologists for their common benefit and for scientific discussions and demonstrations; and to disseminate knowledge of the principles and practice of pathology in relation to medicine by such means as may be thought fit.

2. To consider and advise as to any course of study and technical training and to diffuse any information calculated to promote and ensure the fitness of persons desirous of qualifying for membership of the College...'.

No doubt these wordy assertions were also designed to impress and please, but within 2 years, those not already members of the College discovered that they had to pass an unpleasant examination before they could enter the fold and be certified as specialist pathologists.

For the first 10 years of the College's existence, the actual dissemination of the knowledge of the principles and practice of pathology was assured merely by the presentation of papers and workshops at annual meetings. These did not fulfill the requirements or demands of members and so, in 1967, the Board of Education was created to look after the problem of continuing education. This Board considered several methods, and eventually decided to concentrate its efforts in anatomic pathology on what were called 'surveys'. In fact, these were, and still are, nothing more than histopathology microscopic slide seminars in which participants voluntarily return their anonymous answers for marking and assessment. The first was held in 1968 under the direction of a Western Australian, Professor R. E. J. ten Seldam, who said: 'The aim of the Survey was not to provide a set of slides of rare or unusual cases, but in a broader spectrum to test not only the diagnostic ability of the participants, but also the way in which, as consultants, they would answer the questions asked. To whet the appetite of the more sophisticated amongst us, a few rarities were included'. You can see that despite its name, the philosophy of the newly created Board of Education was virtually the same as that of the Board of Censors; the emphasis once again was on testing rather than teaching.

College members who had indicated their wish to participate in the Survey by responding to a circular and by paying a fee in the order of $A20.00 were posted 12 haematoxylin and eosin-stained histological sections with accompanying brief clinical histories. They were asked a number of questions, and had to return their answers anonymously. Answers were marked; correct diagnoses were counted; and the results were published in a printed booklet distributed at the 1968 Annual College Meeting held in Melbourne, where Professor ten Seldam gave a brief illustrated verbal presentation of the cases and answers. The 12 cases chosen were: carcinoid tumour, ileum; glioblastoma multiforme, left occipital lobe; liposarcoma, soft tissues, right thigh; pneumocystis carinii pneumonia; silica granuloma, skin of chin; giant follicular lymphoma, cervical lymph nodes; granulosa cell carcinoma, left ovary; mesonephroma, left ovary; granulomatous

colitis; adenoid cystic carcinoma, submandibular salivary gland; nodular sclerosing Hodgkin's disease, cervical lymph node; and sarcoidosis of skeletal muscle. The collection undoubtedly tested diagnostic ability over a broad spectrum,
but after looking at the sections, one sophisticated pathologist remarked that his
appetite for rarities was satiated. That year 17% scored less than 7 out of 12, and
only 61% correctly diagnosed 9 or more of the 12 sections.

Similar types of cases were selected through the next 7 years, the main
restricting factors being the availability of enough tissue to prepare 200 sections,
and the adequacy of follow-up information. The general format of each report
was similar to the one you have today in your satchel on pages 47 to 76 of the
blue booklet entitled 'The Royal College of Pathologists of Australia, Board of
Education, 1975, Reports of Surveys, Sydney Meeting, October 1975, in con-
junction with the 9th World Congress, World Association of Societies of Pathology' and edited by H. Kronenberg and K. A. Rickard. Copies of previous
reports are available in large medical libraries.

The work involved in the organisation and preparation of such a national
undertaking was considerable, and almost immediately became too much for
one man to do in his spare time; so, for the next 3 years, Professor ten Seldam
was assisted by Dr. L. R. Finlay Jones and in 1969 by Dr. J. B. Blackwell as well.
From 1972 to 1975, the survey was arranged in turn by the South Australians,
Dr. E. G. Hardy, Dr. D. W. Henderson, Dr. A. Holoyda and Dr. Pauline Hall,
each with assistance from myself. Next year a group of Queenslanders headed by
Dr. Robin Cooke will be the organisers.

So far, the participants have been asked one or more of the following questions: What is the diagnosis? Is further information required? Should more
blocks be cut? Are special stains required? Would you tell the clinician more
than the diagnosis? What is your place of residence (i.e. particular Australian
State, New Zealand or Overseas)? What is your degree of training (specialist
histopathologist, general pathologist, trainee)? Is this answer a joint effort or the
work of one pathologist? Do you have any comments? Can you provide any
literature references to this condition?

Some of the questions encouraged participants to submit ambiguous, incomprehensible or multiple answers; others, such as the question on special stains,
invited extended lists of procedures that most pathologists in practice would not
perform and which were too numerous and involved to be included in a concise
report. As a result, the diagnosis was the only question to be asked in all the
surveys, and in 1975, the organisers would only consider the first submitted
answer.

The number of sets distributed and the number of answers received each year
can be seen in Figure 1, which shows that approximately 100 sets were distribut-

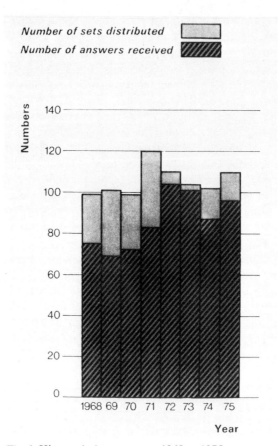

Fig. 1. Histopathology surveys, 1968 to 1975.

ed every year except 1971, when the number increased to 120. The reason for the increase is not known, but it is of interest to note that a 100% increase in cost of the survey in 1974 was not associated with a large decrease in the number of participants. Perhaps most sets were purchased by institutions rather than by individuals. Fewer answers were returned in 1974 than in the two preceding years, possibly because there were 24 cases in that set (so that participants would get their money's worth for the 100% cost increase). No doubt, some who normally supplied answers for 12 cases did not have the time or energy to examine and seriously consider 24 cases. In any event, our generosity was counterproductive. The larger number of answers received in the years 1972 to 1975 when compared to the period 1968 to 1971 was probably due to two factors: in the later years, participants were encouraged to answer as individuals rather than as a group; and secondly, reminder notices with the closing date for receipt of answers were posted to participants in 1972, 1973 and 1974.

Figure 2 shows the percentage each year of participants scoring less than a generally acceptable score. It should be noted that the scores for 1974 and 1975 are not strictly comparable with those of previous years because there were 24 slides in the 1974 set and 15 in 1975. One can see that participants did worst in 1971, when 39% scored less than 7 out of 12, and best in 1975, when only 12% scored less than 8 out of 15.

The diagnoses of the 1971 cases were: cellular intracanalicular fibroadenoma, breast (cystosarcoma phylloides); isolated myocarditis; inflammatory fibroid polyp, small bowel; cytomegalic inclusion disease, kidney; benign osteoblastoma, vertebra; congenital syphilis, liver; peritonitis arenosa, ileum; synovial chondromatosis, hip joint; acinic cell tumour, parotid gland; acute fatty liver of pregnancy; and Pindborg tumour, mandible. No doubt the organisers supposed that these cases would not be any more 'difficult' than those of 1968, but this supposition was not borne out by the answers.

During the entire 8 years, only 1 section, from a case of temporal arteritis, was correctly diagnosed by all; at the opposite extreme, none were answered incorrectly by everyone. The lowest scores were not recorded for all years, but in 1968 1 person scored 1 out of 12. On 7 occasions, diseases were repeated in subsequent

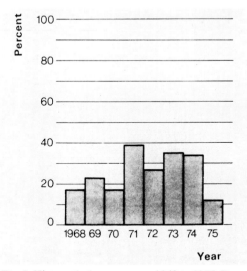

Fig. 2. Histopathology surveys, 1968 to 1975. Percentage of participants scoring less than 7/12 or 14/24 or 8/15.

surveys: on 4 of these, participants performed better at the second attempt; on 2 they performed worse; while on the seventh the same percentage returned acceptable answers each time. The biggest change in scores on repeated cases was from 64% correct to 5% correct in the cases of bizarre smooth muscle tumours. Many questioned the correctness of the organisers' diagnosis of the second case; and even today, the correct diagnosis of that 'leiomyoblastoma' is still being argued.

A comparison of the scores of specialist histopathologists, general pathologists, trainees and pathology laboratories submitting joint effort answers is of interest. Specialists produced the best scores for 2 years; laboratories submitting joint answers fared best 1 year; in another year specialist answers and joint answers were equally good; and on 1 occasion, the trainees did better than all the rest. Shortly after that, the organisers ceased recording the status or experience of participants. At the opposite end of the scale, the trainees performed worst of all groups on 3 occasions, while the generally trained pathologists performed worst twice in the 5 years that these figures were kept.

TABLE 1

Diseases misdiagnosed by more than 50% of participants

Diagnosis	Year	% correct answers
Mesonephroma, ovary	1968	49
Sarcoidosis, voluntary muscle	1968	38
Tuberculous endometritis and Arias-Stella reaction	1969	38
Alveolar rhabdomyosarcoma, chest wall	1970	11
Parosteal osteosarcoma, femur	1970	19
Krabbe's disease, brain	1970	49
Peritonitis arenosa, ileum	1971	7
Synovial chondromatosis, hip joint	1971	48
Acute fatty liver of pregnancy	1971	46
Inverted papilloma, bladder	1972	45
Lymphangiomyoma, retroperitoneum	1972	32
Thorotrast-induced hepatoma	1973	33
Haemangioma, voluntary muscle	1974	21
Subacute sclerosing panencephalitis	1974	35
Congenital 'fibrosarcoma' chest wall	1974	23
Bizarre smooth muscle tumour, mesentery	1974	5
Lymphomatoid granulomatosis, lung	1974	46
Cholegranulomatous lymphadenitis, portal lymph node	1974	44
Metastatic adenocarcinoma in small bowel	1975	31

Table 1 lists the diseases misdiagnosed by more than 50% of participants. In 2 of these, less than 10% of answers were correct, but, as pointed out earlier, the organisers may have made a mistake with the bizarre smooth muscle tumour, and in the case of peritonitis arenosa the organisers rejected the term 'fibroma' by which the condition is known in the American literature (Wood, 1967).

All the conditions listed in Table 1 are rare; so rare in fact that no pathologists, except those in the largest laboratories, would be likely to see another example in practice more frequently than once every 5 years. One could argue that such an inordinately high concentration of rare diseases in a series of 12 or 15 cases must throw doubt on the reliability of these surveys as true measures of the overall quality of Australian and New Zealand surgical pathology reports. Doubtless it explains why so few correctly diagnosed all cases (Fig. 3).

In attempting to assess participants' overall performances, one should consider a number of variables that might have affected scores. The most obvious is the 'ability' of the participants, but other factors almost certainly played an important part. A few of these would have been: (1) the participant's previous pathology training; (2) the time spent studying the slides and answering the

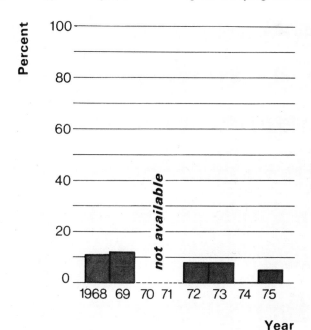

Fig. 3. Histopathology surveys 1968 to 1975. Percentage of participants with all diagnoses correct.

questions; (3) the number of sections in the series; (4) the availability of an adequate medical library; (5) the type of cases selected; (6) the technical inadequacies of the sections distributed (sometimes all sections were not fairly representative of the lesion); (7) the stringency of the marking; and (8) the organisers' own knowledge of pathology. Of these, some details of the participants' training and the number of cases in the sets have been recorded in the published reports, but information concerning the other factors was either not requested or not recorded, or was too subjective to be easily measured.

Despite these shortcomings, the Board of Education of the Royal College of Pathologists of Australia has established a kind of periodic test that is reasonably popular with both qualified and trainee pathologists. Fairly detailed records of this test are kept, published and distributed, and some yearly comparisons can be drawn. Scores are probably affected by many factors. It is difficult to see how all variables could all be eliminated without resorting to examination room-type supervision of participants. Nevertheless, it is probable that the knowledge of those who looked at the slides and read the reports was improved by the surveys, excepting perhaps those few who diagnosed all cases correctly.

We in Australia can therefore justly claim to be pursuing excellence, but I have no doubt that the pursuit would be hotter if we were to concentrate more on the teaching than the testing. As a first step in this direction, the Board of Education intends to collect and make available for loan teaching slide sets similar to those distributed free of charge in the United States. Doubtlessly they will be associated with improved scores, particularly if organisers select for surveys cases that have previously been used in teaching slide sets. If we pursue such a policy, I believe these surveys will become a reasonable test of pathologists' willingness and ability to continue their education, but the relationship of the scores to pathologists' excellence will still be debatable.

Acknowledgements

I would like to thank all the previous survey organisers as well as Dr. A. Palmer, Dr. E. Hirst, Dr. H. Kronenberg and Dr. K. Rickard, who have spent so much time and effort selecting cases and preparing and checking the reports. Thanks are also due to the very large number of Australian and New Zealand pathologists who have contributed cases from which the final few were chosen, and to Miss S. Eden, who typed this manuscript.

Reference

Wood, D. A. (1967): In: *Tumours of the Intestines,* pp. 27, 30, 31. Armed Forces Institute of Pathology, Washington, D.C.

Automated SNOMED coding and the automated autopsy reporting system

G. E. Gantner Jr.

Department of Forensic and Environmental Pathology,
St. Louis University School of Medicine, St. Louis, Mo., U.S.A.

Present routines for capturing autopsy data usually involve narrative dictation, typing of reports and listing of diagnoses by organ system or by sequence of events. The development of the Systematized Nomenclature of Pathology (SNOP) has greatly aided in the capture and retrieval of diagnostic data. It provides a broad data-base approach to the analysis of cases, adding appreciably to the quality of retrieved material. More recently the College of American Pathologists along with a large advisory group from other medical specialties has extended the SNOP concept to all of medicine in the Systematized Nomenclature of Medicine (SNOMED). Even this extended nomenclature, however, is greatly enriched if it can be supplemented by adding demographic data (e.g. age, sex, etc.) and weights and measures (e.g. height, heart weight). The author has designed a system which will capture descriptive and other data from the prosector by providing suitable lists of descriptive statements for each organ from which one or more suitable choices are made. A record of each choice is kept and the system then branches to the next appropriate 'screen' of up to 10 alternative choices according to a predetermined logic. This system is known as the Automated Autopsy Reporting System (hereafter referred to in this text as AARS) and it provides the prosector with an efficient, personalized way of capturing his own autopsy data and providing a quick autopsy narrative and diagnosis list (less than 15 minutes). In addition it automatically assigns the all-important diagnostic codes for 95-98% of all stated and implied diagnoses.

Division of labor

Demographic data can be input by a secretary or morgue personnel. Clothing descriptions of routine cases can similarly be captured. The prosector is free to start his own input with items peculiar to his specialty of pathology and starts with the external medical description. Moving along from screen to screen, information is presented in a 'conversational' mode with little chance of forgetting data, using improper formats or spending time on questions which the system can be programmed to ignore based upon earlier responses. Following the prosector's input (less than 10 minutes actual time) additional enriching information can be added by chemists, toxicologists, bacteriologists and other members of the professional team having something to do with that particular case. In popular terms each member 'does his own thing'.

Basic concepts

Working much like the classical automated history techniques, the system provides the 'questions', the prosector the answers. However, certain important linkages have been added which greatly enrich the AARS process. Each choice or descriptor has associated with it:

1. A descriptor number for future record and reference;
2. An associated sentence or sentence fragment for later insertion into a standard autopsy 'paragraph';
3. An associated diagnostic equivalent, if appropriate, for the diagnostic listing;
4. An associated diagnostic code, where appropriate, e.g. SNOP, SNOMED (SNDO or ICDA where a concept can be coded);
5. A screen 'jump routine', logic-driven to avoid looking at unnecessary screens.

Insertion of unlimited freeform narrative is described below.

Statement type

In the list above the phrase 'where appropriate' appears repeatedly. It became evident early in development that descriptive statements could be categorized into five levels based on the expressed or implied diagnoses contained in the statement. These types are as follows:

A. Contains a diagnosis established by the gross examination alone;
B. Contains a diagnosis requiring microscopic confirmation;
C. Secondary (incidental) diagnoses;
D. Observations requiring explanations (if possible);
E. All purely descriptive and normality statements.

This list of five categories covers all possible statements used in the AARS system. Statement types, A, B, C, or D elicit a separate page listing. Type E, being descriptive, only appears in the printed paragraphs, not in the diagnostic listings.

A typical CRT screen for heart size is shown in Figure 1. In the example choice 1 obviously is a statement of normality. On the other hand, choice 3 states a diagnosis. This latter will later print on the diagnosis list with its diagnostic codes.

How it works

As screens are presented to the prosector he chooses one or more of the descriptions (depending upon screen type). The software then branches to the next screen along a predetermined path which may skip one or more upcoming screens. Each choice is stored for each screen so that the coded message in storage looks like this:

2694, 2711-420, 2721, 2731, 2753, 2771-25-4, 2802, 2903, 2931-13-10-11.4-9, 2974, 2983, 2991, 2979, 2982, 3041, 3081, 3097

where 2694 is the heading 'Heart' and 2711-420 indicates that screen 271 is the heart weight and choice 1 (i.e. 2711) is an actually weighed, not estimated, heart

(2751)	=	The size and contours of the heart are normal.
(2752)	=	The heart is enlarged.
(2753)	=	The left ventricle is hypertrophied.
(2754)	=	The right ventricle is hypertrophied.
(2755)	=	Both ventricles are hypertrophied.
(2756)	=	The heart appears greatly dilated, probably as an agonal event.

Fig. 1. Screen 275: heart size.

weight. The weight in this case was 420 g. Other screens show their choices and measurement entries: e.g. 272 choice 1, 273 choice 1, 275 choice 3 and screen 277 choice 1 (= actual ruler measurement) and the measures -25 and -4 standing for millimeter thicknesses of the left and right ventricles respectively (see Fig. 2 for narrative equivalents).

It may be mentioned that since the 'jump' routine is completely structured only choices and weights and measures need to be stored. Thus the coded heart description can actually be stored as:

4, 1-420, 1, 1, 3, 1-25-4, 2, 3, 1-13-10-11.4-9, 4, 3, 1, 9, 2, 1, 1, 7

or even

41-4201131-25-4231-13-10-11.4-943192117.

Assuming the computer program, screen detail and 'jump' instructions which were actually used at the time of the terminal entry are permanently available, the entire narrative etc. can be reconstructed and reprinted exactly as originally input. Subsequent changes in the narrative wording to a later developmental form will not interfere. However any change in jump routines will make the use of the above short symbolic form unpredictable in reconstruction of the narrative.

As each organ 'set' is completed, a subprogram takes the screen choices and weights and measures and prints out the organ heading and narrative descrip-

(2694)	=	Heart:
(2711-420)	=	The heart weighs 420 g.
(2721)	=	The surface is smooth, glistening and transparent.
(2731)	=	The wall is of normal consistency.
(2753)	=	The left ventricle is hypertrophied.
(2771-25-4)	=	The left ventricular wall measures 25 mm and the right 4 mm in thickness.
(2802)	=	The endocardium, cardiac valves and chamber are normal except
(2903)	=	That the aortic valve shows marked arteriosclerosis with calcification.
(2931-13)	=	The tricuspid valve measures 13.0 cm in circumference,
(-10-)	=	The pulmonary valve 10.0 cm,
(-11.4-)	=	The mitral valve 11.4 cm,
(-9)	=	And the aortic valve circumference 9.0 cm.
(2974)	=	The anterior descending branch of the left coronary artery
(2983)	=	Shows arteriosclerotic narrowing up to 75% obstruction.
(2991-2979)	=	The other coronary vessels are
(2982)	=	Patent but show some atheromatous streaks.
(2992, 3041)	=	The cut surface of the heart is of the usual reddish brown color.
(3081)	=	The left ventricular wall
(3097)	=	Shows diffuse whitish scar tissue.

Fig. 2. Equivalent descriptive statements.

tion paragraph. Since the screen choices are almost infinitely variable in combinations an important part of the software program directs the printing of the narrative in proper sequence and with appropriate line length (see Fig. 3). This printing data is actually stored in a computer memory buffer until the printer itself is available.

After all of the screens have been viewed and selections made, the printer prints out the narrative descriptive paragraphs from the buffer and turns to the next task. Diagnostic lists are printed in their appropriate categories (A-D) along with the appropriate diagnostic code selected (preferably SNOMED). Figure 4 shows the diagnostic list generated from the heart choices above. Note that they are in order of acquisition and are not necessarily in order of importance. Hierarchical ranking requires an additional important step which will be described below.

Figure 5 shows a very complex narrative description in which structured descriptors have been supplemented by detailed freeform narrative. This can be as rich as the prosector desires. It may be input via the terminal keyboard or captured by dictation with the screen number indicated. The secretary simply types the screen number and the narrative into the terminal and the program does the rest. One additional chore is created by the use of freeform descriptions and that is the necessity of visually and manually extracting stated and implied diagnoses and their corresponding SNOMED codes. In order to simplify this

---

Heart: The surface is smooth, glistening and transparent. The wall is of normal consistency. The left ventricle is hypertrophied. The left ventricular wall measures 25 mm and the right 4 mm in thickness. The endocardium, cardiac valves and chamber are normal except that the aortic valve is calcified. The tricuspid valve measures 13.0 cm in circumference, the pulmonary valve 10.0 cm, the mitral valve 11.4 cm, and the aortic valve circumference 9.0 cm. The anterior descending branch of the left coronary artery shows arteriosclerotic narrowing up to 75% obstruction. The other coronary vessels are patent but show some atheromatous streaks. The cut surface of the heart is of the usual reddish brown color. The left ventricular wall shows diffuse whitish scar tissue.

Fig. 3. Narrative paragraph as actually printed for the gross report.

	SNOP	
(1) Left ventricular hypertrophy	T3260M7200	(from choice 2753)
(2) Calcified aortic valve	T3900M3610	(from choice 2903)
(3) Ant. descending branch left Coronary atherosclerosis	T4311M5210	(from 2974 + 2983)
(4) Left ventricular scar, diffuse	T3260M5475	(from 3081 + 3097)

Fig. 4. Provisional gross anatomic diagnosis.

The heart weighs 440 g. The surface is smooth, glistening and transparent. The surface also shows some epicardial hemorrhages. The wall is of normal consistency and there is a normal amount of subepicardial fat tissue present. There are three recently sutured incisions in the left atrium. A pacemaker lead enters the superior vena cava. It is covered with fibrous tissue. Both ventricles are hypertrophied. The left ventricular wall measures 18 mm and the right 4 mm. The endocardium and chambers are not remarkable. The aortic valve has been replaced by a Starr-Edwards valve which is functionally intact. The circumference of the tricuspid valve is 105 mm, the pulmonary 80 mm, the mitral 80 mm, and the aortic 80 mm. The mitral valve shows moderate arteriosclerosis. The right coronary artery is found to have a chronic, complete atherosclerotic obstruction. This occupies a segment 1 cm long located between 2 cm and 3 cm from the orifice. There is a functional vein graft running from a point beyond the obstruction and in an area only 50% occluded. This connects to the aorta 2.5 cm above the aortic valve. The other coronary vessels are found to have atheromatous obstruction up to 95%. The cut surface of the myocardium is the normal reddish brown color. The posterior portion of the left ventricle and the posterior portion of the interventricular septum show diffuse old scar tissue.

Fig. 5. Complex narrative description.

(A) Diagnoses firmly established by gross examination alone

1	Myocardial hypertrophy	T3300M7200
2	Arteriosclerosis mitral valve	T3800M5200
3	Atherosclerotic occlusion right coronary artery	T4320M5210
4	Atherosclerosis coronary arteries, severe	T4300M5210
5	Diffuse old infarct posterior left ventricle	T3260M5475
6	Diffuse old infarct posterior septum	T3241M5475

Narrative additions to text

(2721) There are three recently sutured incisions in the left atrium. A pacemaker lead enters the superior vena cava. It is covered with fibrous tissue.

(2801) The aortic valve has been replaced by a Starr-Edwards valve which is functionally intact.

(2971) There is a functional vein graft running from a point beyond the obstruction and in an area only 50% occluded. This connects to the aorta 2.5 cm above the aortic valve.

Additional diagnoses (enter via (add DX) routine)

7	Pacemaker	T3200M1550
8	Aortic stenosis	T3900M3610
9	Excision aortic valve	T3900M1520
10	Starr-Edwards replacement for aortic valve	T3900M3211
11	Vein-bypass-aorta to rt. coronary artery	T4320M1563
		T4210M1563

Fig. 6. Provisional gross anatomical diagnoses.

the program actually prints out these 'narrative additions to text' separately (as well as within the paragraph). As a separate operation the prosector can quickly scan and extract diagnoses and add their SNOMED codes. These are subsequently added through a terminal via the 'Add Dx' routine. Line numbers are assigned in sequence with those automatically extracted. This process is illustrated in Figure 6.

The 'hierarchical arrangement' screen is now called and by a special subprogram the diagnoses are rearranged by inserting their line numbers into tab positions in a primary, secondary and tertiary arrangement as illustrated in Figure 7. The final diagnostic list and codes properly sequenced and arranged are now printed (Fig. 8) for the final time. New diagnoses from the microscopic process are handled identically. Suspected diagnoses eliminated by the microscopic or other procedures or tests can also be eliminated during the screen entry procedure by simply ignoring the insertion of the line number.

In a special study 100 consecutive hospital autopsy cases were analyzed. 95% of all diagnoses were automatically captured despite numerous freeform narrative inserts. Thus, only 1 diagnosis in 20 necessitated using the SNOP code book – a real plus for 'coders who hate to code'. An additional 100 medico-legal

Primary	Secondary	Tertiary
*		
8		
	9,10,1	
4		
	3	
		5,6,11
	7	
2		

Fig. 7. Worksheet (or CRT screen): hierarchical arrangement of diagnoses.

1.	Aortic stenosis	T3900M3610
	A. Excision aortic valve	T3900M1520
	B. Starr-Edwards replacement for aortic valve	T3900M3211
	C. Myocardial hypertrophy	T3200M7200
2.	Atherosclerosis coronary arteries, severe	T4300M5210
	A. Atherosclerotic occlusion right coronary artery	T4320M5210
	(1) Diffuse old infarct posterior left ventricle	T3260M5475
	(2) Diffuse old infarct posterior septum	T3241M5475
	B. Pacemaker	
3.	Arteriosclerosis mitral valve	T3800M5200

Fig. 8. Final anatomical diagnoses.

cases from the St. Louis County Medical Examiner's office fared even better, with 98.5% of all diagnoses captured by the automated aspects of the program. This confirms the fact that medico-legal autopsies are (as they should be) even more highly structured than hospital cases. While freeform descriptive inserts were very extensively used in the medico-legal cases, the additional diagnostic content of these descriptions was quite minimal. It must be admitted that, since the author is a practicing forensic pathologist who performs numerous autopsies, the program routines have been designed to address data capture in these areas especially thoroughly. This fact is 'transparent' to prosectors of hospital autopsies since the routines jump over unneeded material. The prosector views a question set tailor-made to his particular case.

St. Louis County Medical Examiner
Name: Thomas, Judith A.
Address: 5605 Filmore
Age: 27 years
Race: Caucasian
Sex: Female

Medical examiner's number: 75-427
Prosector: Gantner
Postmortem exam: 9/25/75 at 11 A.M.
Injury (best estimate) 9/25/75 at 8:30 A.M.

Administrative data 9/25/75
Death: at 8:30 a.m.
(known rather precisely from reports)
Occupation: Housewife
Status: Married
Medical Examiner's case
History suggests death by: accident
Death certificate by: County Medical Examiner
Investigator: Ernst
Depth of investigation: pathologist
Body brought from: public place
Agency: County Police
Disposition: burial

External examination: body weight estimated at 180 lb. Body length: 70 inches. The state of preservation is good. Postmortem rigidity of the jaws is absent, of the neck absent, of the arms absent, and of the legs absent. There is a normal state of nutrition. Cyanosis is absent. There is no peripheral edema present.

Personal hygiene is good. No operative scars are present. There is a crush injury of the chest. There are lacerations of the forehead, orbital region and lids, lips, nose, left upper arm, left forearm, right upper arm, right forearm, left thigh and right lower extremity. There are multiple fractures of the ribs. There are fractures of the right tibia, right fibula, left humerus, left radius, left ulna, right maxilla, left maxilla, left zygoma, and right frontal bone.

Fig. 9. Demographic data and external examination.

Portions of a medico-legal case emphasizing the demographic data and the external part of the exam with a subsequent diagnostic list and diagnostic codes are shown in Figures 9 and 10. In the illustrations multiple equivalent diagnostic codes are printed together for comparison. In actual practice the prosector selects the desired diagnostic code prior to printout. If two coded sets are required two separate lists are requested. The program automatically SNOMED 'codes' if a code is not specified.

Figure 10 also illustrates the arrangement on the first printing of diagnostic statement type into: (A) diagnoses firmly established by gross exam alone; (B) diagnoses requiring microscopic confirmation; (C) secondary diagnoses; and (D) observations needing explanation. Type E, which includes all purely descriptive and normal statements, do not print in this listing for obvious reasons.

Appendix 1 shows a complete first printing of a gross examination and diagnostic listing with codes. Reading of the narrative in this case will provide the reader with the 'flavor' of the screen choices in additional organ systems. Note that the diagnosis on line 14 lists a 'probable' bronchopneumonia which will be later deleted if not confirmed by the slides. In designing the system the author decided that it was far easier to use an educated guess and predict a diagnosis,

(A) Diagnoses firmly established by gross exam alone

		SNOP	SNOMED
1	Chest crush injury	TY210M1481	TY2100M1040
2	Forehead laceration	TY011M1440	TY0110M1440
3	Orbital region and lids laceration	TY048M1440	TY0480M1440
4	Lips laceration	T5210M1440	T52000M1440
5	Nose laceration	T2110M1440	T21000M1440
6	Left upper arm laceration	TY820M1440	TY8200M1440
7	Left forearm laceration	TY850M1440	TY8500M1440
8	Right upper arm laceration	TY820M1440	TY8200M1440
9	Right forearm laceration	TY850M1440	TY8500M1440
10	Left thigh laceration	TY910M1440	TY9100M1440
11	Right lower extremity laceration	TY900M1440	TY9010M1440
12	Ribs multiple fractures	T1133M1260	T11330M1280
13	Right tibia fracture	T1173M1200	T11730M1200

(B)   Diagnoses requiring microscopic confirmation: none

(C)   Secondary diagnoses: None

(D)   Observations needing explanation: none

Fig. 10. Diagnostic list for the same case.

even though it would possibly be deleted later, than to add it later (easy in itself) and also look up the code number (a little more work). From the tactical standpoint it is probably easier to capture (predict) any probable diagnosis since it is so easily ignored and deleted in the hierarchical rearrangement process. Even mutually exclusive possibilities could *all* be listed with only the confirmed ones surviving to the final printing and computer storage. In the illustration only a single additional procedural diagnosis would need to be added and coded from the SNOMED 'Procedure' field. A similar tactical design approach will be employed with developments currently underway. Thus a subprogram will consider heart weight, left ventricular thickness and other parameters and automatically check an internal parameter table and by algorithm 'decide' whether the diagnosis of 'left ventricular hypertrophy' is justified or not. If challenged by the prosector the program could print or display its logic, its detailed parameter table and the literature or 'standards commission' reference.

Are the statements too personalized?

While the statements are in the author-designer's own words it must be appreciated that the program works on concepts and is independent of individual expression. Thus the concept 'left ventricular hypertrophy' is really an intellectual one which is expressible in English, French or any other medically complete written language. Likewise, the symbolic language of SNOP, using T-3260, M-7200 or SNOMED, using T-32600, M-7100, is conceptually equivalent to the English language 'left ventricular hypertrophy'. The described programs are exactly like SNOP and SNOMED in that the concept is what the computer sees, manipulates, stores and prints. Dr. Roger Cote, University of Sherbrooke, Quebec, Canada, has designed and uses a unique program which can read SNOP (SNOMED) diagnoses in either French or English, then store the code and printout in either French or English as required in that bilingual community. The author's AARS is similar to this concept and stores even the narrative statements in a universal (internal and unseen) program-recognizable code. Any narrative statement in the AARS dictionary can be replaced by any other conceptually equivalent narrative statement in personalized or stylized words and in any written language. A new system user can go over the statement dictionary and replace any or all statements with his own preferred expressions so that it will report in his own personalized way. Thus one of the outstanding advantages of the symbolic nomenclature SNOMED – universality and transferability of language – can be realized for narratives too. Another feature which makes SNOMED powerful is also utilized. SNOMED breaks concept expressions into fundamental components of anatomy, abnormality at that site, causative agent, etc. by use of multiple coding 'fields'. Thus an inflammation (M) may occur at any site (T). The initially attractive economy of combining site and disease into a single code (ICDA) irrevocably trades off significant and important detail which can only be obtained by returning to the source document. SNOMED's fields more closely match the natural language sentence structure so that a sentence in the AARS can actually be constructed from multiple screens, each fragment carrying along its own SNOMED code. This would be virtually impossible with combined site-disease codes.

Does the system require an elaborate computer?

The system was originally designed and debugged via pencil-type data forms, Hallerith-type punch cards, and a batch mode computer. An input device is required which will present the total choices, capture those selected and present them to the computer for processing. This could include teaching machines with punched paper tape, mark-sensed cards and sheets, key-punched cards, various keyboards and other terminals including (ideally) a cathode ray tube system. The main computer program is written in Fortran IV, and requires approximately 16,000 bytes of core memory utilizing 1000 Fortran statements. The dictionaries are much larger and contain over 150,000 characters. However the dictionaries are dealt with sequentially, raising the possibility of using various magnetic tape systems, even cassettes. Prosector time at the CRT is usually less than 10 minutes and processing more like 15 seconds of central processor time. The total number of screens is 300, with the shortest path through the routines being 125 screens.

Storage formats and retrieval

Only the choices are stored, along with weights and measures, freeform narrative, inserts and the final hierarchical rearrangement of diagnoses. While the diagnostic codes could be reestablished by passing the storage numbers back through the dictionary programs, it is much more efficient to store the codes themselves separately. The small amount of additional storage space required provides a set of case labels which can be efficiently sorted by the computer when searching for cases without going into the detail of the case until it has been identified. Cases may even be referenced by 'inverting' the diagnostic code file (i.e. placing all similar codes together along with their case numbers). Inverted files provide highly efficient retrieval. In my experience all large data bases should be referenced from inverted files. (Private collections of certain types of cases of personal interest constitute examples of inverted file storage.) Retrieval can be made by any group of parameters as specified in Boolean terminology utilizing a special retrieval program. Mixed searches of demographic, diagnostic and descriptive concepts can be made. Freeform narrative is retrievable as such but, being unstructured, it is not suitable for further machine analysis.

Additional applications

Once data has been captured and stored in machine-readable form, the applications to which they may be put are limited only by the creativity of the human mind. The author uses the AARS approach for capture and retrieval of his own hospital and medico-legal case loads. In the medico-legal applications systematized capture of investigative data is enriching the autopsy data and adding new scientific possibilities never before pursued in this area. Environmental pathology can be studied by supplementing the autopsy data with specialized environmental, occupational, smoking, dietary and home environmental histories which use the same programs but with different screens, different dictionaries, different jump routines and a different handling of the assembled data. For student prosectors or history-takers the classical computer-assisted instruction benefits can be realized. Specialized tumor registry questions are easily addressed and can be specialized for individual cancer types.

Summary and conclusions

A system has been described which captures and organizes autopsy data by providing suitable descriptive statements, a branching logic and links these statements with levels of diagnostic terminology. Diagnostic codes are automatically assigned for 95-98% of diagnoses in routine and medico-legal autopsies. Freeform narrative inserts are accommodated easily, requiring only the manual look-up of the diagnostic codes. The system allows the vast richness of autopsy data to be computer-accessed, processed and utilized for a myriad of practical scientific purposes with minimal outlay of additional time, effort and financial resources. The AARS system is a useful extension and companion to the SNOMED diagnostic codes. It constitutes a powerful new tool for the capture and utilization of medical data and gives added support to the usefulness and importance of the multifield SNOMED approach to the national and international handling of detailed medical information.

APPENDIX 1. Complete first printing of a gross examination and diagnostic listing with codes.

St. Louis County Hospital

Name: Logan, Emma

Autopsy number: 75-465
Prosector: Dr. Gantner

Age: 76 years
Race: Caucasian
Sex: Female

Postmortem exam: 9/25/75 at 1:30 P.M.
Death: 9/25/75 at 1:00 P.M.

Administrative data:
Marital status: Never married
History suggests death due to natural causes
Death certificate by: private physician

External examination: Body weight estimated at 130 lb. the state of preservation is good. The body is slender. Lividity is unfixed and is primarily found on the anterior body surfaces and upper portions of the body. Cyanosis is absent. There is no peripheral edema present. Personal hygiene is good. The hair is gray and this apparently represents the natural color. The hair is worn in a long female style. The body hair is of normal female distribution. The pupils are round, regular, equal and somewhat dilated. The irides are hazel. There has been a cataract removed on the right. The gums are edentulous and dentures accompany the body. The female breasts are atrophic. The external genitalia are normal. Operative scars are present. This is in the right upper abdominal region. There are no injuries or fractures present.

Body cavities: The body is opened with the usual Y incision. The abdominal fat layer measures 40 mm in thickness. The anterior musculature and subcutaneous region are not remarkable. The peritoneal cavity shows no free fluid or adhesions. The right pleural cavity shows no fluid or adhesions. The left pleural cavity shows no fluid but adhesions are present. The left pleural adhesions are moderate. The pericardial cavity contains fluid estimated at 10 ml. The fluid is serous.

Neck organs: The soft tissue of the neck shows focal areas of hemorrhage. The thyroid gland weighs 32 g. The thyroid gland is enlarged. The parathyroids are not identified.

Heart: The heart weighs 510 g. The surface is smooth, glistening and transparent. The wall is of normal consistency. The subepicardial fat tissue is increased in amount. The heart is enlarged. The left ventricular wall measures 26 mm and the right 6 mm. The endocardium is normal. The tricuspid valve shows moderate arteriosclerosis, the mitral valve shows marked arteriosclerosis, and the aortic valve shows marked arteriosclerosis. The coronary arteries are normal throughout. The cut surface of the myocardium is of the usual reddish brown color. The aorta shows moderate atherosclerosis. The systemic arteries are in general normal.

Lungs: The lungs together weigh 1650 g. They show congestion and edema. The lungs are free of any injuries. The color of the lung surface is pink. The dependent portions of both lungs show a granular change suggesting bronchopneumonia. The air passages contain purulent material. The process involves the bronchial system in general. The pulmonary arteries are free of emboli, thrombi and other gross lesions.

Liver: The liver weighs 1650 g. It is tan in color and of moderate firmness. The capsule is smooth and glistening. The cut surface shows increased fibrous tissue.

Biliary tract: The gallbladder has been surgically removed. All biliary channels are patent and free of gross abnormality.

Pancreas: The pancreas is not remarkable. The surface is tan in color. The consistency is normal.

Gastrointestinal tract: The entire gastrointestinal tract is examined and found to be normal.

Spleen: The spleen weighs 290 g. It shows marked congestion but is otherwise normal.

Lymphatic system: The lymph nodes are free of inflammation and malignancy.

Bone marrow: The bone marrow is normal.

Adrenals: The adrenals are well supplied with lipoid material and are free of hemorrhage, inflammation, and primary and secondary neoplasms. The medulla is not remarkable.

Kidneys: The kidneys together weigh 390 g. The kidneys are essentially identical in gross findings. The capsule of each kidney strips with ease to reveal a normally smooth surface. The surface is the usual reddish brown color. The cortex averages 10 mm in thickness. The corticomedullary demarcation is distinct. There are no abnormalities of the cut surface of the kidneys. The renal pelves and ureters are not remarkable. No stones are present.

Bladder: The bladder contains an estimated 30 ml of urine. The urine is clear and yellow. No stones are present. The bladder wall is normal.

Female genital system: The uterus is not grossly remarkable. The myometrium is normal throughout. The single intramural leiomyoma measures 15 mm. Both tubes and ovaries are normal for the age of the patient. The vagina is not remarkable. The vulva is unremarkable.

Central nervous system: (Permission to examine the brain was specifically denied in this case).

Provisional gross anatomic diagnoses

A) Diagnoses firmly established by gross examination alone

		SNOP	SNOMED
1	Left pleural adhesions, moderate	T2920M4824	T29200M4924
2	Hemorrhages neck	T0324M3850	T03240M3700
3	Thyroid enlargement	T9600M7200	T96000M7100
4	Cardiomegaly	T3200M7200	T32000M7100
5	Arteriosclerosis tricuspid valve	T3600M5200	T36000M5200
6	Arteriosclerosis mitral valve	T3800M5200	T38000M5200
7	Arteriosclerosis aortic valve	T3900M5200	T39000M5200
8	Coronary arteries atherosclerosis	T4300M5210	T43000M5210
9	Aorta, moderate atherosclerosis	T4200M5210	T42000M5210
10	Pulmonary congestion	T2800M3810	T28000M3610
	Pulmonary edema	T2800M3840	T28000M3650
11	Cirrhosis liver	T5600M4850	T56000M4950
12	Spleen, marked congestion	T0700M3810	T07000M3610
13	Intramural leiomyoma	T8200M8890	T82000M88900

B) Diagnoses requiring microscopic confirmation

14   Dependent portions lungs bronchopneumonia T2812M4001   T28120M4001

C) Secondary diagnoses

15	Edentulism		
16	Atrophic breasts	T0400M7100	T04000M5800
17	Hydropericardium	T3X00M3830	T3X200M3630
18	Cholecystectomy	T5700M1520	T57000M1502

D) Observations needing explanation

None

Narrative additions to text
19   (from # 0841) there has been a cataract
      removed on the right

APPENDIX 2

Automated Autopsy / Time-Shared

Data Base Management Requirements
    1.0 Autopsy Input Code (AIC)
    2.0 Hierarchically Ordered Diagnoses (HOD)
    3.0 Critical Autopsy Parameters (CAP)
    4.0 Population Model Definitions (PMD)

Report Generation Requirements
    1.0 Unit Autopsy Reports
        1.1 Narrative Report
        1.2 Diagnoses Report
        1.3 Critical Parameters Report
    2.0 Population Wide Reports
        2.1 Population Parameter Analyses
            2.1.1 Tabular Presentation
            2.1.2 Static Graphical Presentation
            2.1.3 Dynamic Graphical Presentation
        2.2 Population Parameter Prediction
            2.2.1 Tabular Presentation
            2.2.2 Static Graphical Presentation
            2.2.3 Dynamic Graphical Presentation
        2.3 Population Model Simulation Studies

The problems involved in world-wide standardized evaluation of dissection material

W. Jacob

Pathologisches Institut, University of Heidelberg,
Federal Republic of Germany

Why standardize the evaluation of dissection material throughout the whole world? Given the variety in methods of acquiring and treating dissection material, such an idea seems utopian. All over the world a great number of autopsies are made daily. Epidemiological evaluation of these autopsies is impossible as long as definite, standardized methods of dissection are lacking.

The aims of epidemiological pathology go beyond the range of geographical pathology. Epidemiological pathology is a systematic supplement to clinical epidemiology in its later development, i.e. a differentiated statistical analysis of pathoanatomical organic changes in the whole cadaver, insofar as the examination of such a cadaver is within the scope of definite clinical-epidemiological inquiry. Examples of suitable topics would be epidemics caused by man such as arteriosclerosis and cancer.

Epidemiological pathology has a wider scope than geographical pathology. Geographical pathology determines the frequency of occurrence of certain diseases in different countries under various climatic, economic and sociological (i.e. ecological) conditions. It draws conclusions as to the etiology and pathogenesis, and, in general, the mode of spread and the character of certain infections and other diseases, e.g. metabolic diseases. The aim of epidemiological pathology is to complete and extend this basis by a vertical extension of the statistical evaluation of autopsy findings. It is concerned not only with the frequency of occurrence of a certain disease in a certain area, but also with the various dimensions and categories of the disease process. It tries to get an idea of the effective conditions of the disease process by adequate statistical analysis of the individual dissection findings and the appropriate clinical data, the socio-anamnestic data and the individual findings.

Figure 1 shows that a disease should not only be seen in terms of the organic findings, but also in the context of the pathogenetic influences of the whole human environment which affect the diseased organ. Figure 2 shows the environmental factors involved. This scheme was largely devised by Mrs. Ellinor McDonald (M.D. Anderson Hospital, Houston, Texas) for the epidemiological research of cancer.

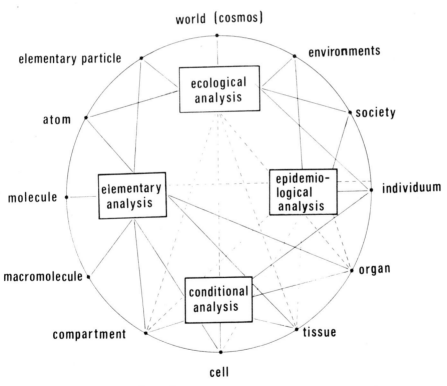

Fig. 1. Factors affecting a diseased organ.

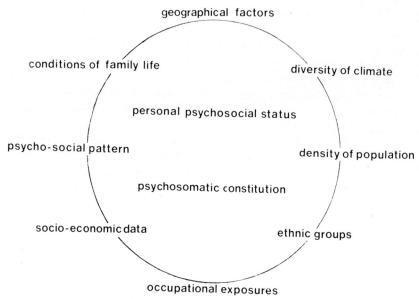

Fig. 2. Environmental factors.

The homeostasis of the bioorganism – regardless of where it starts – is sensitively disturbed and impaired at one or several points. The rules of 19th century pathology are still valid. Virchow's definition reads: 'disease is life under changed conditions with the character of danger'. The scheme presented here is not at all new. The 27-year-old Virchow recognised a social-medical concept in the hippocratic manner in his report on the upper Silesian typhus epidemic. He was not only concerned with the organic findings and the clinical course of the disease, but also with the total ecological human condition. This is exactly the aim and the contribution of epidemiological pathology.

In order to be able to practise epidemiological pathology on a broad basis, we need standardized, i.e. comparable, diagnoses and statements. Such a demand in the area of dissection pathology is difficult to meet. The observations of qualified pathologists vary according to their special preference for a particular organ, corresponding to their scientific interests. This leads to special, detailed diagnoses. The scientific and practical interest, which is the basis of an autopsy, often determines the standard of the findings and diagnoses. A complete scientifically evaluated dissection makes quite different demands in terms of single macroscopic and microscopic examinations than, for example, a routine dissection, a partial dissection or a simple inspection of organs for the purpose of confirming a clinical diagnosis. In other words, we cannot expect that in the different pathological institutes of the world the same dissection techniques will be practised or that the evaluation of results will meet the same standards.

There are practical difficulties. The use of dissection findings as the basis of the pathological-anatomical diagnosis depends in the first place on the execution of dissection and on further examinations of the dissection material.

Obligatory standards can be developed for the technical execution of autopsies and for the histological examination of dissection material. It is more difficult to relate the clinical scientific enquiry connected with the single autopsy to the aims of a standardized protocol or dissection diagnosis. As soon as more complicated statements of fact have to be explained patho-anatomically, e.g. the results of an accident or illness, the examination of single organs or definite topographic and pathological organ references come after the practical scientific problems.

The identification of a focus, e.g. a hidden source of infection, can cause great difficulties and may involve an enormous investment of dissection technique. The scientific, clinical and practical interest of a comparative examination of different forms of carcinoma and its metastatic spread can make it useful to follow the traces of cancer as far as the most remote regions of a lymph gland.

The systematic examination of topologically different distribution patterns with certain factors of risk of arteriosclerosis can make it necessary to perform a detailed examination at different points in the arterial system. The search for a primary tumor or multilocular tumors may completely confuse the routine practice of a dissection.

The simultaneous occurrence of different disease lesions in an organ of a cadaver and the statistical evaluation of primary and secondary findings is a second important factor in epidemiological pathology. Exhaustive, in-depth evaluation of the dissection material should be the aim, and is essential for scientifically based epidemiological pathology.

These aims are bound to meet with practical difficulties: we cannot expect a pathology institute which is handicapped in personnel and equipment to reach the same standard as, for instance, the Armed Forces Institute of Pathology in Washington, to give just one famous example. On the other hand, it is important to establish standards so that epidemiological pathologists can use dissection material not only from the major scientific institutes but also from other institutes all over the world.

My suggestion is to form 6 standard classes, A-F, as follows.

Class A includes a large scientific section distinguished by:

1. Highly differentiated macroscopic investigation findings and a description of all important visual observations made at autopsy.

2. Highly differentiated, precise and complete definition and work-up of the dissection diagnosis.

3. Exhaustive histological examination of all organs and all important regions of the body.

4. Use of different stains.

5. Histochemical examinations.

6. Electronmicroscopic examinations.

7. Bacteriology.

8. Additional biochemical examinations.

9. Photographic presentation of important and interesting findings.

10. Thorough documentation of findings and computer data processing.

11. Record-linked biographic anamnestic, social-anamnestic and clinical findings and pathoanatomical data.

Class B. The formalized dissection record provides a basis for a systematically epidemiological coverage of pathoanatomical dissection findings. It is suitable for use in large university institutes and autopsy departments, but also in smaller departments, and especially when larger amounts of dissection material are being worked up. The protocol can also be evaluated from different points of view if regular histological examinations of the important organs take place.

Class C. A formalized dissection record or diagnosis which considers and comprises the main findings of the autopsy. In general 5-6 organs will be histologically examined. Their weights will be registered.

Class D. Part dissection of one (or several) body cavities for post-mortem interpretation of clinical diagnoses with histological examinations of individual pathoanatomical findings.

Class E. This protocol includes only the dissection findings of a single organ with or without histology for the approximate interpretation of a clinical picture that is still uncertain.

Class F. Inspection of one or several body cavities to confirm diagnoses pathoanatomically (macroscopically).

Classification into standard classes makes it possible to agree on world standards and improve the bases of epidemiological pathology. The advantages are: (1) dissection findings in classes A and B can be investigated individually and analyzed either scientifically or epidemiologically; (2) dissection findings in the same classes are comparable.

For classes A and B one can rely on consistent and thorough interpretation of the findings in all dissections. These findings can also be systematically scientifically examined for certain single findings or statistically analyzed for epidemiology.

Class C comprises the established routine dissection. It can also be used within certain limits for scientific inquiry and epidemiological examination. Dissection protocols in class C can be used for epidemiological studies based on large numbers of autopsy findings generally.

Standard classes D and E belong to the category of emergency dissections for immediate post-mortem clarification of a clinically unclear picture. These classes are not suitable for systematic evaluation for epidemiological studies, unless they are related to clinical findings. However, these standard classes are very important in clinical diagnosis and therapy, and, within limits, observations on the frequency of certain diseases in the scope of geographical pathology.

If standardized protocols are used, we know immediately to what extent pathoanatomical material of the same class can be compared and epidemiologically evaluated. The lowest standard class used for epidemiological evaluation – being the weakest link in the chain of pathoanatomical investigations – determines the evaluation of pathoanatomical findings for epidemiology.

Protocols in classes A, B and C can be evaluated epidemiologically, provided that the terms of class C are used and not the terms of class A or B.

For very specific scientific questioning special autopsy concepts must be drawn up to ensure consistency in examinations of different organs or body regions. This applies to all long-term prospective epidemiological projects in which pathology plays a role, e.g. examinations in epidemiological research on arteriosclerosis or cancer.

What should be the next practical step? My suggestion is to obtain, collect and document, according to the suggested standard classes, information about dissection techniques and findings in different areas of the world. Would it be possible to divide such a study into regional areas and to form regional centres whose task it would be to register and collect information on the dissection techniques used and to document dissection findings at different institutes? At a later stage these centres could also grant educational aid for the performance, standardization and epidemiological evaluation of dissection material.

A suggestion for a first concrete attempt at world-wide comparison, documentation and evaluation of dissection material was originated by Professor Doerr, Director of the Institute of Pathology in Heidelberg. The recommendation was to exchange dissection protocols from three or four large institutes over the whole world, to collect them at a central point, evaluate them by the suggested standard classes and compare the epidemiologically important data (dissection diagnoses, dissection protocols) over about one year. If we could compare dissection material from large institutes in for example Japan, the U.S.A., South Africa, Canada and South America, we would have a better idea of possible future steps.

Coding should be based on the latest edition of SNOMED. We are now able

TABLE 1

Comparison of results using a standardized and a free-text protocol

	Data missing		Data completely present		Data incomplete		Data to be presumed from the context		Not checked		Extra	
	No.	%	No.	%	No.	%	No.	%	No.	%	No.	%
Standardized protocol	253	4.9	4299	84.3	299	6.0	133	2.6	58	1.1	58	1.1
Free (dictated) protocol	2215	43.5	2503	49.0	252	5.0	94	1.8	36	0.7	—	

From Brüst et al., 1974, *Virchows Arch. path. Anat., 364,* 1.

to document such dissection diagnoses and protocols and to data-process them. The formalized protocol worked up by W. W. Höpker at our institute has already been introduced at several German pathology institutes.

Table 1 shows a comparison between the data noted using a free (dictated) dissection protocol and a standardized protocol. In the standardized protocol only 4.9% of the data normally expected in a dissection protocol have been omitted. In the free (dictated) protocol this percentage was 43.5.

The data were complete in 84.3% of dissections made using a standardized protocol, as compared to 49% using a free (dictated) protocol. The percentage of incomplete data was about the same in both protocols: 5% in a free (dictated) protocol and 6% in the standardized protocol.

In the standardized protocols 2% of data had to be assumed from the context; in the free (dictated) protocol this figure was 1.8%. The percentage of unchecked data was 1.1 in the standardized protocol and 0.7 in the free (dictated) protocol. More than 4000 dissections have been statistically evaluated.

Author index